Why Hospitals Should FLY

The Ultimate Flight Plan to Patient Safety and Quality Care

By JOHN J. NANCE, JD

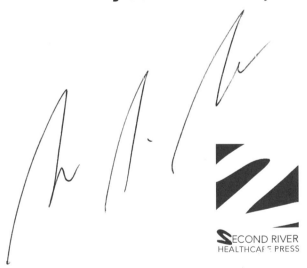

SECOND RIVER
HEALTHCARE PRESS

WHY HOSPITALS SHOULD FLY
The Ultimate Flight Plan to Patient Safety and Quality Care

Second River Healthcare Press
26 C Shawnee Way
Bozeman, MT 59715
Phone (406) 586-8775 | FAX (406) 586-5672

Senior Editor & Cover Design: Christopher R. Jackson
Editors: Lee Reeder & John J. Byrnes, MD
Cover Art: Roger Schillerstrom
Author Photograph: Bridgitte Krupke
Typesetting/Composition: Neuhaus/Tyrrell Graphic Design

Nance, John   Why Hospitals Should Fly: The Ultimate Flight Plan to Patient Safety and Quality Care / John J. Nance, JD

ISBN-10: 0-9743860-5-7 (hard cover)
ISBN-10: 0-9743860-6-5 (soft cover)

ISBN-13: 978-0-9743860-5-8 (hard cover)
ISBN-13: 978-0-9743860-6-5 (soft cover)

1. Patient safety   2. Quality care   3. Health services administration

Library of Congress Control Number: 2007940532

First Printing   April 2008

Second River Healthcare Press books are available at special quantity discounts.

Please call for information at: (406) 586-8775 or order from the websites:
www.SecondRiverHealthcare.com or **www.WhyHospitalsShouldFly.com**

TABLE OF CONTENTS

DEDICATION

To Kathleen Bartholomew, RN, MN, whose enlightened understanding of human nature has guided this book and its grateful author as effectively as her tireless efforts to elevate the profession of nursing.

AUTHOR'S NOTE

How can it be that in 2008, a checked bag on an airline flight is still exponentially safer than a patient in an American hospital?[1] Simply put, one industry has learned the realities of what it takes to make a human system safe, and the other has not.

So what *does* it take to dramatically improve patient safety and service quality? It takes a host of new and different (and sometimes radical) methods centered on supporting the people on the front lines — those who actually take care of the patient. It takes a hospital like the one in this story: St. Michael's.

St. Michael's itself is fictional, but it is specifically designed to show how the ideal healthcare environment would look and feel. Are all the methods and ideas and organizational characteristics in use at St. Michael's largely in use in real institutions? Not yet, though many are in the process of being adopted, and some are already producing wonderful results. In fact, I encourage you to visit our website (WhyHospitalsShouldFly.com) for updates over the next few years on which institutions are making such changes and where you can get help and advice in following their examples.

But the bottom line is this: What St. Michael's represents is an achievable paradigm, and if we can't imagine what constitutes truly safe and collegial hospitals, we can't build them.

John J. Nance, JD
Seattle, April 2008

FOREWORD

In 1957 Ayn Rand first asked the question, who is John Galt in her famous opus *Atlas Shrugged*. More than half a century later the world is still intrigued by the John Galt character and his inventiveness, renegade personality and ability to shatter the status quo. Today, I am moved to ask, who is John Nance with the same attendant power of that original 1957 question.

I am confident that readers of this terrific new book will be transformed as though visiting Galt's Gulch in *Atlas Shrugged* when they complete their journey to the fictitious St. Michael's Hospital in the suburbs of Denver, Colorado. Nance's character, Dr. Will Jenkins, is akin to a first time visitor to Galt's Gulch, eerily also thought to be in the suburbs of Denver, Colorado. Dr. Jenkins stumbles upon a unique place, expertly described by Nance, that has somehow managed to turn traditional hospital culture upside-down and inside-out as it moves the safety agenda forward. Readers will be transfixed by the characters Nance has created who populate St. Michael's Hospital — leaders like Dr. Jack Silverman, the CEO, himself a former busy surgeon and nurses like Patti Miller, currently working on her Ph.D. in safety.

I can't think of anyone active at the national scene in quality and safety in healthcare who could have written a book like this one. Nance is a formidable character in real life, as a decorated military pilot, attorney, television celebrity and global airline safety expert. In addition, he is a recognized award-winning writer who knows how to tell a story and create lasting and impressive characters. In this book, Nance has brought together all of his formidable skills to create a story full of drama, pride, motivation and outright wonder. He takes a seemingly bland subject like improving the safety of medical care and tells a story that is heartfelt and compelling. I can truly say that Nance's book reads like a novel and I simply couldn't put it down.

As Dr. Will Jenkins makes his exploratory trip to St. Michael's we begin to viscerally appreciate the challenges that St. Michael's has faced and the characters literally come alive to illustrate important themes like crew resource management, cultural change, and process improvement, in order to create a so-called high-reliability organization. All of this mind numbing jargon, leaps out of the pages as the characters illustrate the human dimension of these new terms in ways that only Nance could have created.

Having seen Nance in action numerous times and witnessed his power over audiences large and small, sophisticated and novice, the pages of this book conjure up those memories for me. I can see him in my mind's eye working the crowd, pushing, pushing and getting results. In some way, Dr. Will Jenkins is *everyone* sitting in an audience listening to Nance. Dr. Jenkins goes about his exploratory work at St. Michael's with an open mind and slowly his dramatic conversion occurs. Jenkins is in the audience at every Nance presentation.

Who is John Galt? We may never really know for sure and the question is as compelling today as it was in 1957. After reading this book, I think we will be able to ask the question, who is John Nance and what has he wrought? No one will be the same after a visit to St. Michael's. No one will view a medical error and simply shrug that this is how it has to be. Every healthcare leader needs to read this book and press it into the hands of each stakeholder in their local environment. Every medical student needs to read this book as a prerequisite for graduation, and finally, every surviving family member who's loved ones were victims of a medical error could take heart in this new book and explore St. Michael's in more detail. For me, St. Michael's will always be Galt's Gulch and John Nance is John Galt.

David B. Nash, MD, MBA
The Dr. Raymond C. & Doris N. Grandon Professor & Chairman
Department of Health Policy
Jefferson Medical College
Philadelphia, Pennsylvania

INTRODUCTION

When one contemplates the progress in improving patient safety over the past decade, several apparently contradictory facts leap out: We know a lot about how to prevent injuries, and the efforts to improve have been substantial, yet too many people still die from medical mistakes.

The facts are irrefutable. Despite the "wakeup call" from the Institute of Medicine (IOM) in 1999, tens of thousands of patients still die unnecessarily and hundreds of thousands are injured by medical mistakes every year. It is currently estimated by the CDC, for example, that as many as 90,000 people die from hospital acquired infections alone. At least 10 percent of patients admitted to hospitals are injured by things going wrong in their care.

To be sure, some progress has been made. The Institute for Healthcare Improvement's (IHI) *100,000 Lives Campaign* of several years ago had a major impact in motivating thousands of hospitals to implement several tested safe practices. And, undoubtedly, over 100,000 lives were saved. But many more are still being lost unnecessarily to medical mistakes.

The theory is sound. We know how to prevent medical injuries. The IOM report that got so much attention also made a clear and unambiguous observation: It's not bad people, it's bad systems. Fix those systems! More than a half-century of thought, experimentation, and hard work in cognitive psychology, human factors engineering, and several high-hazard fields, most notably aviation, underlie that recommendation. Systems failures cause human failures. Fix the systems if you want to stop medical mistakes and injuries.

The efforts to fix systems have been enormous. Since the IOM report, there has been a steady crescendo of increasing development, testing and implementation of new safe practices by hospitals throughout the country. At the urging of IHI, professional organizations, and the Agency for Health Research and Quality

(AHRQ), as well as in response to increasing requirements from the Joint Commission, hospitals have been striving to implement safe practices such as identity checking, time-outs, hand hygiene programs, protocols for procedures and dozens of other practices. Most hospitals have designated patient safety officers and quality improvement teams who are trying to make changes.

Yet, the progress has been painfully slow. Why? Why, with all this effort and commitment, do we have so little to show for all of this? Why are hospitals still incredibly hazardous places to enter — worse, perhaps than ever? Why has it come to pass that all major organizations now recommend — not permit, recommend — that patients always have someone with them while in the hospital?

The answers are perhaps as varied as the questions one asks, but a common theme that comes through in discussions with caregivers on the front lines and those who think a great deal about patient safety, is our failure to change our culture. What we have not done, they say, is create a "culture of safety," as has been done so impressively in other industries, such as commercial aviation, nuclear power and chemical manufacturing. These "high-reliability organizations" are intrinsically hazardous enterprises that have succeeded in becoming (amazingly!) safe.

Worse, the culture of health care is not only unsafe, it is incredibly dysfunctional. Though the culture of each health care organization is unique, they all suffer many of the same disabilities that have, so far, effectively stymied progress: An authoritarian structure that devalues many workers, lack of a sense of personal accountability, autonomous functioning and major barriers to effective communication.

What is a culture of safety? Pretty much the opposite! Books have been written on the subject, and every expert has his or her own specific definition. But an underlying theme, a common denominator, is teamwork, founded on an open, supportive, mutually reinforcing, dedicated relationship among all participants. Much more is required, of course: Sensitivity to hazard, sense of personal responsibility, attitudes of awareness and risk, sense of personal responsibility and more. But those attitudes, that type of teamwork and those types of relationships are rarely found in health care organizations.

It is John Nance's contention, which I fully share, that we will not achieve safe health care, regardless of how many new safe practices we implement, unless and until we change to that type of culture: Until we value what everyone brings to the patient encounter and rededicate ourselves to a new way of "practicing" our professions.

The changes required are enormous. Why haven't health care leaders, so far, been up to the challenge? In part, perhaps because they haven't recognized that the problem is one of relationships, not of know-how or resources. In part, also, perhaps because of lack of experience, either personal or vicarious, that provides them with an emotional understanding of practice in this type of culture. They don't *really* understand what it would be like, much less the kind of changes it will take to get there.

John Nance provides that experience and understanding. Framed as fiction, but heavily laced with lessons from the real world, the story of St Michael's transformation to a culture of safety shows how it can be done. There are no bleeding hearts in this story. The protagonists, both those who have changed and the skeptical visitor, are all hard-nosed realists, people who work on the front lines of medicine where egos are big, tradition is strong, change is difficult and the stakes are immense. They know it is difficult, and they have scars to show for it. But more importantly, they show it is possible. You want to know what a culture of safety in health care is like? Start reading.

Lucian L. Leape, MD
Harvard School of Public Health

CHAPTER ONE

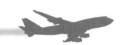

The 240-bed not-for-profit hospital hardly looked like the site of a revolution, quiet or otherwise. But the praise that had drawn Dr. Will Jenkins to this suburb of Denver, Colorado, had been unequivocal. St. Michael's, he was told, was the locus of a renaissance.

Designed in the '50s, he concluded, noting the green metal trim of the exterior as he turned into the parking lot. But if it was pedestrian on the outside, somehow on the inside the staff and leadership of St. Michael's Memorial had managed a miracle: three years with no sentinel events, no patient safety incidents, patient and staff satisfaction scores off the chart on the high side, and a mortality rate so low it was attracting a flood of visitors from the far corners of health care.

Will parked the rental car and killed the engine as he looked at the ordinary brick and mortar exterior, squat and undistinguished under the cobalt blue canopy of a June sky. To the west, the front range of the Rockies stood high and imposing like a frosted pastry, still covered with a mantle of late spring snow. He'd barely noticed the snow during the drive from the airport, so intent was his concentration on the telephone exchange that had lured him here.

As promised, Dr. Jack Silverman, the CEO, was waiting for him in the lobby with the no-nonsense air of a busy surgeon. Silverman led the way to his office and plopped himself behind the desk, fixing his medical visitor with a penetrating gaze as Will settled into the offered chair.

"Will," he began, "I'm aware that what we've done here is so unusual a growing tide of people want to come study us to death, but frankly, I don't have much time to spend explaining it. Over the next three days I'll spend some time showing you how different our culture is and how we figured it out, but the rest is up to you. Now, you and I are very much alike in that we're two doctors who've gravitated over time into administration, but we're still clinicians at heart, and fixing things — especially patients — is a shared passion. So I think I know what you're after, and I've prepared a reading list for you, plus a folder full of internal papers and explanations. You'll also have a chance to meet and talk with some of our key people, but if you want to get the same results in another hospital, you'll have to start with your own massive culture change."

"I understand," Jenkins answered.

"No, I doubt you do," Silverman said as he came forward, his elbows on the cluttered desk. "Now, this is where we differ in terms of experience. No offense intended, Will, but I doubt that you or even 5 percent of the doctors and hospital leaders out there have the ability to speak the same language we now speak. Here's the problem: Everyone who comes here thinks they can just cherry-pick a few of the changed attitudes they observe, drop them into a business-as-usual hospital model, and all will be well, but that doesn't even begin to work. In fact, there's no way I could overemphasize how important a point this is: What we've accomplished here cannot be duplicated by just putting *some* of our programs in place. What's required is a complete reprogramming of the medical delivery culture. And I do mean a complete cultural overhaul."

"Well, I *do* understand that the central element of your success was the adoption of the aviation model," Jenkins said.

Silverman began with a chuckle that rose to a full laugh as he shook his head. "Yes, the aviation model is the key to the same extent that intubation is the key to a heart-lung transplant — a required, pivotal component, true, but only part of the story. Will, those great procedural things from aviation are just the tip of the iceberg. CRM, for instance — crew resource management — is an incredibly effective way of getting leaders to involve subordinates and listen to them as real team members. It revolutionized the airline cockpit by getting rid of the unresponsive, maverick captains who refused to listen to anyone, and it's a principle that's helped us considerably here. But the real brilliance of what aerospace has discovered about human safety systems comes more from a subtle understanding of how to transform an imperfect, mistake-ridden, high-risk human culture into a culture of colleagues who actually can achieve near perfect safety.

"Perfect safety, by the way, doesn't mean eliminating all mistakes. It means structuring a system that expects and safely deals with mistakes, both the type that can do immediate harm and those that can kill slowly — such as failing to lower someone's critical cholesterol levels over time. Dealing with failures effectively is the essence of a high-reliability organization. The kicker is that even though they discovered it and pioneered the process of taking a dangerous enterprise to HRO status, few aviation leaders even today fully understand how they've achieved such incredible levels of safety. By contrast, most major healthcare leaders *do* understand it, even though we have yet to achieve HRO status. There's an excellent paper out about that very point I've got for you in the packet.[2] But back to the airline leaders. It was almost tragic/comic, when I began this quest, because I started by sitting down with several airline chairmen, only to find that not one of them really understood even the basics of the human revolution that has made their industry so amazingly safe. I had to do some very deep research of my own to learn how to crack the code. Once I realized that safety and quality depend on having unified teams of like-minded people willing to put all normal human and professional differences aside to achieve a common goal, the theory began to come together. Applying that theory and actually changing us was a different story, of course. That was, and is, a matter of hard and sustained work built around the clearly stated common goal that everything we do here is done for the best interests of the patient."

"You're telling me the airlines don't even understand why they've been so successful?"

"They understood the tactics — the courses and training and principles of cooperating in the cockpit — but what they'd forgotten, or never realized, was that none of those tactics would have worked if they hadn't changed their culture. Now, *Boeing* understood it."

"Boeing?"

"Boeing took everything their airline customers knew about the tactics of creating teamwork and clear communication in the cockpit and combined it with a brilliant stroke of common sense to create a breakthrough example," Silverman explained. "In Boeing's case, the strategy was both incredibly simple and incredibly difficult, because it involved changing a hierarchical, hidebound culture that had evolved over nearly a century. There was real arrogance in the idea that aeronautical engineers were too good to dirty their hands by dealing directly with mere customers, or even with those who cut the metal to build the airplanes they designed. In many respects, those senior engineers were acting exactly the way we physicians act. But Boeing's leaders, and especially a gifted engineer and leader named Alan Mulally, crafted a new concept called "Working Together" to kickoff the design of a critical new jetliner that became the Boeing 777. Now, Working Together is similar to a thousand phrases we've used in health care, but Mulally made it the battle cry of cultural change, and he went for no less than a cultural renaissance. The whole approach was opposite to the traditional way they'd done things, and it's wildly different from, and almost assaultive to, the way we've always done things in medicine. But I can tell you that it's the only method I've ever experienced that can take a gaggle of independent, ego-driven, mutually-suspicious professional humans and turn them into a real team truly dedicated to the same common purpose."

"Are you sure you're running a hospital here?" Jenkins laughed.

"Not like one you've ever experienced, I'll bet. For instance, Will, one of the things we do here is study every failure and near-miss to the point that all of us become truly eager to share our mistakes for the common good. And, while none of us like to dwell on our failures, we constantly discuss the fact that we owe it to those we've injured or killed in the past to never forget that we have a duty to fix the system that failed them. I imagine as a former hospital CEO you've got a few sad stories of your own."

The memory of the disaster that had propelled Will here filled his mind for the briefest of moments, but it was enough to contract his stomach again. He pushed the feeling away and pulled out a small, silver object and gestured to it. "May I run my digital voice recorder? I don't want to miss a word of this."

Getting to his feet, Silverman nodded, well aware of his younger colleague's ashen expression and suspecting what had probably prompted it. After all, he thought to himself, Jenkins had been far too relentless in getting this appointment to be driven by mere academic interest.

"You can run the recorder, or even bring in a camera crew, but until you've spent some time watching us, you haven't a prayer of understanding how it works. You got the suggested schedule, right?"

"Yes. Spend the rest of today observing..."

"Well, tonight at least. First the ER, then some clinical settings. Jack Silverman's patented three-day course."

"And, if I wasn't serious enough to want to learn..."

"Right, you'd never put up with this curriculum. Weeds out the insincere."

Will followed Silverman into the corridor, his mind unable to set aside the memory that had been triggered moments before. Never mind that years had passed, it was still fresh and painful and mortifying.

Never in his 16 years as a physician had Will Jenkins felt as helpless and depressed as he had on that terrible night in 2003. Of course, as a doctor, he'd lost patients before without knowing why, and as a CEO he'd presided over many more tragedies. But this one was different, and he had mishandled virtually every aspect of it.

For the three years immediately preceding that night — from the first day he'd been appointed CEO — he'd worked tirelessly and with growing confidence to build an entirely new era of quality and accountability into the suburban community hospital near Portland, Oregon. The earthshaking 1999 report of the Institute of Medicine had shocked him profoundly. The title of the IOM's seminal work was *To Err is Human*, and its premise was nothing less than bringing the previously shunned subject of medical error into the glaring light of public and professional scrutiny. But it was the part of the report that said American hospitals were killing just under 100,000 patients annually from avoidable medical mistakes that had moved Will to face down his board to get the necessary money to start changing things. He had dived in fearlessly by hiring consultants, holding meetings, and even bringing in an energetic group of former fighter pilots to train his physicians in OR teamwork. He'd mandated the use of "time-outs" in the hospital's surgical suites (although the rumors persisted that the surgeons were ignoring the directive), and threatened to pull privileges for physicians who failed to attend his training sessions. He'd even weathered a furious lawsuit by one of the physician groups and forced a change in the medical bylaws to give him the unquestioned authority to throw out a physician who refused to comply, and he'd used much of his credibility with the board in the process. His staff members and even the charge nurses had been Six-Sigmaed, Lean-Meaned, Studered, Joint Commissioned, trained in Toyota's methods, and lectured by a dizzying variety of experts. They'd filled notebooks with the six steps to this and the seven deadly problems to that, and his reports to the board of everyone's determination to "zero out" professional mistakes had been glowing and full of promise. It might be true, he'd told his board members, that up to 96,000 patients were being killed by mistakes in America's hospitals, but being killed by avoidable medical errors was no longer a probability at Memorial.

And then the roof fell in, and despite all his efforts, yet another completely avoidable medical mistake in one terrible evening took the life of a young patient, garnered the undivided attention and excoriation of the media, and effectively canceled everything they'd accomplished. After two years of public shame, litigation, and a ruinous verdict against his hospital, he could bear it no longer. Will's embarrassed resignation had followed. It seemed the only honorable course of action, but it hurt to have had it accepted so quickly by the panicked board. Chastened and filled with self-doubt, he had packed up his wife and three kids and found a different state, doubting that he'd ever be competent to run a hospital again.

For years after, it haunted him, as did the obvious inability of the medical community to put a substantial dent in the death rates from medical mistakes that were clearly caused by a combination of human errors and flawed systems. The thought was always with him that somehow he'd missed something in applying all the accepted solutions at his former hospital. Even as he resumed an uninteresting private practice, he found himself frequenting the nearest medical library, determined to figure out how he had failed.

The research left him amazed at how many thousands of hospital leaders across the nation had apparently tried to handle the challenges of medical mistakes the same way he had, and with the same disheartening results. Patient safety, he realized belatedly, had been treated like a specific disease for which a specific vaccine could be formulated. But by 2005, two things had become painfully apparent. Despite six long years of sound and fury in health care about the emergency need to improve patient safety, just as many patients seemed to be dying as the result of medical mistakes. Equally disheartening, many uncounted others had lost significant quality of life to wrong-site disasters, unnecessary surgeries, and a horror-writer's laundry list of other heartrending human tragedies.

He searched for, but could never find, the evidence that would suggest that the mass of American hospitals had changed for the better, though he heard rumors from time-to-time about various institutions that were taking maverick action and making significant inroads. The field was awash with hospital executives just as puzzled and frustrated as he, all of them wondering why the "fixes" they tried had barely made a dent in the unconscionable rate of accidental deaths and injuries. Yet month-after-month physicians were still cutting on the wrong appendage or the wrong patient, good nurses were still grabbing lethal doses of the wrong medications, and across the nation many of the procedures, such as surgical time-outs and other double-checking methods were failing from lack of standardization.

If there was a "magic bullet" to use on the specter of medical errors, Will had lost faith in its existence, until the small article about a Denver area hospital caught his attention.

It was a nondescript facility called St. Michael's Memorial, the writer said, and it was being hailed as providing a true glimmer of light in an otherwise dark landscape of poor progress. Apparently, where others were failing wholesale across the nation, St. Michael's was succeeding by standing routine medical expectations on their head. It wasn't the only hospital to show patient safety improvement in the nation by any means, but St. Michael's did seem to be the only institution to have so totally altered the model and the ethos of a modern hospital that it was turning heads.

The author of the article had been amazed at the unheard-of attitude adopted at St. Michael's that no matter what else they did to minimize error, they agreed to adopt an artificial attitude that in every procedure, diagnosis, test, or other professional interaction with their patients, there was still at least a 50-50 chance of something major going wrong. It had nothing to do with proof or national averages or local experience. The hospital-wide presumption was a prophylaxis, and it was applied by everyone in every case universally. "Here," she wrote, "...are the best and the brightest doctors and nurses not only admitting they are capable of making life-threatening mistakes, they've created an entirely new culture that routinely *anticipates* such mistakes, and thereby catches life-threatening mistakes others routinely miss." If there was a precedent for such a complete overhaul in thinking, Will had never encountered it.

In addition, St. Michael's seemed to have created an entirely new definition of what "teamwork" really meant. "The trick," its CEO, who was also a physician, had been quoted as saying, "is understanding that only a special type of teamwork and camaraderie can catch, in time, the types of medical errors a hospital will always generate."

"Catch," not "prevent." The shift in emphasis practically screamed at him from the page, all but mocking the fact that all his efforts as a CEO had centered on prevention. His operative assumption had been that once safety system problems were repaired, errors didn't need to be anticipated because they simply weren't going to happen.

The last quote had rung a bell in his head. "In other words,"

Silverman had said, "what we can accomplish as a team of mutually-respectful and supportive colleagues, checking one another for the common good of keeping our patients safe from unnecessary harm, we could never accomplish working alone."

Will had called Silverman that very afternoon, and now, as he pulled himself from the memory, he saw the senior physician stopping in front of a double-door entry to the emergency department.

"Okay, here's the deal. I'm going to introduce you to the ER staff, and I'm going to get back to my day. What I want you to do is go back to your hotel, have dinner, read some things I've got for you in this envelope, and get back here at 8 p.m. and stay until 1 a.m. I want you to observe, ask questions, take notes, then get some sleep and meet me for a very early breakfast at 7 a.m. tomorrow, ready to tell me what you saw and what it means."

"Sounds like a good plan."

Silverman pushed at the door and stopped, hesitating as he watched Will's face. "You remember the bronze bust of our founder I showed you a minute ago as we passed the lobby? The late Dr. Martin, one of the pioneers of emergency medicine?"

"Yes."

"He's our equivalent of Captain Jacob van Zanten."

"Excuse me?"

"The best and the brightest, and yet he was still all too human. You ever hear of a place called Tenerife and the world's deadliest airline accident that happened there in '77?"

Will was nodding now, embarrassed to have forgotten the name.

"Yes. I've... studied it."

"Well, Dr. Martin had his Tenerife right here in the early '70s, and it killed him. The story is in that folder. Essentially, it was a wrong-site surgery that so devastated him he left practice and died a year later."

"You knew him?"

"He's the reason I carry a stethoscope. He was my grandfather."

CHAPTER TWO

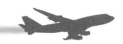

The modest dining room of the mid-level hotel was predictable but blessedly quiet as Will ordered, sipped at a glass of Napa Riesling, and pulled the considerable stack of papers from Jack Silverman's envelope.

On top was the story of the terrible events of March 27, 1977, on the small island of Tenerife in the Atlantic. Several of the consultants Will had retained during his halcyon days as a hospital CEO had routinely taught various aspects of the Tenerife accident, and he'd studied the official accident report himself, missing at first the profound lessons the tragedy held for medicine. He pulled the paper closer and began reading a version he'd never encountered, one drafted by Silverman himself that focused primarily on the captain.

"TENERIFE"

or...

PATIENT SAFETY 101 for St. MICHAEL'S STAFF

As summarized by your CEO, Jack Silverman

The Unthinkable

"Tenerife" was the single accident that changed aviation and the airline business forever. It robbed a generation of senior airline captains of the myth they could avoid serious mistakes by merely the force and effect of their experience, their position and their presumed infallibility. But, in fact, Tenerife has had vastly more to say to the world of human professionals outside aviation than to aviation itself. It has been dramatically effective in reaching the human center of even the most case-hardened and resentful physicians and medical leaders who try to persist in the fiction that they're immune to error and somehow devoid of a need to depend on teams to keep their patients safe.

One of the most profound elements of this tragedy is that the person most responsible was neither a negligent individual, nor a bad person. He was, in effect, the best and the brightest aviation had to offer, and that means he was similar to the best senior surgeon you've ever known or respected. What happened to Captain Jacob van Zanten on March 27, 1977, in Tenerife was in many respects the same scenario that has occurred to so many respected doctors who have accidentally injured or killed a patient. In other words, the human aspects of this story — the lack of communication, the misunderstood words, the pecking order obscuring vital information, and the assumptions not challenged — could have all occurred just as easily in any OR, any ICU, or any ER.

There's one other thing all doctors, nurses, CEOs, pharmacists, dieticians, housekeepers and CFOs need to understand, since medical professionals often try to discount the similarity of cockpit life with life in command of any aspect of medicine: the idea that the dedication and concentration of pilots are somehow different because unlike doctors, their lives are on the line. "It's not the same," health care critics often say, "since pilots fear dying in a crash, while medical people — despite being personally devastated by a medical error that hurt someone — nevertheless usually survive, both personally and professionally."

Not true! In fact, airline captains do NOT fear dying in a crash of their own creation. After all, those cockpits have never killed them before, and commercial flying is almost perfectly safe. What professional pilots fear is making a professional mistake so significant and damaging that the whole world finds out about it. They fear diminishment as accomplished experts in their field. They fear being looked down upon by their peers. They even fear adverse legal action more than they fear dying in a crash. In other words, what they fear is precisely what a doctor or a CEO or a nurse-manager or chief nursing officer fears. We are, in fact, almost identical in our hopes and fears because even if we won't admit it, we sense our fallibility.

Let me put you mentally and emotionally in that 747 cockpit now and walk you through the basic facts of what happened. But, please, think of Captain van Zanten (the guy sitting just in front of the cockpit jump-seat you're occupying) as *Doctor* van Zanten, with the mission ahead of him as nothing more than a routine surgical procedure. Imagine the copilot/first officer as the equivalent of the anesthesiologist, and the second officer/flight engineer as the equivalent of the scrub nurse.

It's just before noon and the single-runway airport on the small island of Tenerife in the Canaries has been saturated with more airplanes than it was designed to handle at one time. Hours before, a botched terrorist explosion at the main island airport of Las Palmas prompted officials to shut down all inbound and outbound flights to the capital of the Canary Islands, leaving nearly a dozen arriving airliners with too little fuel to do anything else but head for an alternate landing on Tenerife. With one small parking area to the west end, and half the taxiways not able to handle the weight of the two Boeing 747s that are among the arriving air force, the physical challenges of landing that many airliners at Tenerife is prodigious, and complicated by the fact that the two tower controllers have very limited ability to speak Aviation English (the required international language of air traffic control).

The weather is not cooperating. Clouds are blowing across the runway more frequently and creating fog-like conditions, and as the afternoon has worn on, the weather has been threatening to ground all the airliners that have sought temporary refuge. With no guarantees on when the main airport at Las Palmas will reopen, the various airline captains have been making difficult decisions on whether to keep everyone aboard for a rapid departure or let them roam around the small terminal, and whether to burden the single fuel truck available for more jet fuel.

In command of a brightly colored blue and white Boeing 747-200 filled with holiday-bound charter passengers headed for Las Palmas is the airline pilot most every airline pilot on the planet aspires to be: Captain Jacob van Zanten, chief pilot of KLM Royal Dutch Airlines, a corporate vice president, the director of safety, the "face" of KLM's recent advertising campaign, and a family man with more than 30 years of near-flawless performance.

Of course, relatively few airline pilots on the planet know of Jacob personally, but younger pilots are well aware of what it takes to reach his position. Many have routinely fantasized about what it would be like to be a chief pilot, a vice president, or a captain so senior that virtually everyone else is of lower rank and lesser experience and capability.

There is also an overall assumption that a man of such great rank and experience has undoubtedly put his last significant mistake behind him. Like the captain of the mythical Starship Enterprise — Captain James T. Kirk — someone in the command position of a Jacob van Zanten is not only officially expected to be perfect, he is widely *presumed* to be perfect. In fact, the universal belief in his omnipotence is supported by the entire culture.

And, of course, perfect people need no advice, but as the hours have ticked by at Tenerife, Jacob himself has been reminded that he is anything but perfect, regardless of his job description. He has already been kicking himself for making two irritating mistakes: Letting his passengers get off the aircraft to go wandering around the airport terminal just before Las Palmas decides to reopen, and ordering too much fuel in an effort to avoid refueling in Las Palmas for the leg back to Amsterdam.

The first mistake has become embarrassingly apparent as he's had to send members of his crew to the terminal to try to round up all the passengers while blocking literally all the other airliners on the ramp. The last to taxi in on arrival, Jacob let himself be parked like the cork in the bottle, blocking all the other diverted airliners. No one can move until he moves, and he can't move until the fueling is completed and his passengers have all been re-boarded.

The second mistake has not only monopolized the single fuel truck, it's made his KLM 747 heavier than it needs to be for takeoff from Tenerife's relatively short runway. And from the position of a senior commander who should make tough decisions look effortless, the whole thing is turning into a very bad day. For a man known for never getting upset, he can feel himself becoming irritated and openly snappy.

There is a third problem lurking in Jacob's consciousness, and it involves two subjects for which he's known to be a taskmaster back in Amsterdam: keeping the operation on schedule, and adhering precisely to crew duty-time limitations. If it takes too long to leave Tenerife, and even if he gets out before the fog shuts down his departure, he might have to delay the leg on to Amsterdam by 12 hours in order to get his crew the required rest. That alone will cost the company over 30,000 dollars in hotel rooms for the inconvenienced outbound charter group, and it will leave the airline one 747 short for the rest of its worldwide schedule. Jacob is well aware the word will get around the pilot group in less than 24 hours, and he'll be living down the embarrassment for a long time to come.

With approximately 10 minutes left before running afoul of the crew duty-time deadline, Jacob finishes the engine start procedures, releases the brakes, and begins following the tower's heavily accented instructions to taxi all the way down the runway and turn around in position to be the first aircraft off.

In the intervening hours, the blowing clouds have become an all but solid fog, and not even the tower controllers can now see the position of the various aircraft they are controlling verbally by radio. Behind KLM, other aircraft are receiving taxi clearances as the controllers work on unsnarling the mess at the west end parking area.

At the east end, Jacob turns the huge Boeing around, straightens the nose wheel for the takeoff roll, and verifies his copilot has finished the checklist.

The first officer/copilot, a very experienced pilot both senior as a copilot and very junior to Jacob, suddenly looks to his left. Shocked, he realizes that Jacob's right hand is moving forward the four thrust levers that control the 50,000 pound thrust, JT-9D Pratt and Whitney engines.

Jacob, he realizes, is starting the takeoff roll. But the copilot knows the tower controller has not issued a takeoff clearance!

Without hesitating, the copilot addresses Jacob, well aware the captain could have him fired.

"Wait, we do not have the clearance yet!"

Jacob van Zanten, the chief pilot, the veteran, for whom the thought of making such a mistake is beyond embarrassing and horrific, now does what uncounted millions of professionals regularly do when confronted with the possibility that someone might think them imperfect: He pulls the throttles back and says; "I know that! Get the clearance."

The copilot, internally shaken, presses his radio transmit switch and asks the tower controller for the first of the two clearances that Jacob has forgotten. The first, known as the Air Traffic Control Clearance, is the set of instructions to fly to Las Palmas. The other is the actual takeoff clearance which will allow KLM to roll the half-million pound aircraft down the runway, accelerating to 142 knots and liftoff.

The Spanish-speaking tower controller begins reading the details of the ATC clearance to the Dutch-speaking crew in heavily accented Aviation English as the copilot begins writing it down.

Ahead of the huge KLM 747 a fuzzy wall of fog is obscuring all but the first white line of the runway centerline. With official visibility barely legal for takeoff and conditions worsening by the minute, the pressure to leave immediately is increasing.

The ATC clearance seems to rattle on forever in Jacob's estimation as he feels the remaining time ticking away. In fact, it takes merely seconds, followed by the copilot's required read-back of the clearance on the radio to make sure he's made no mistakes. As the copilot approaches the end of the read-back using the notes he's copied down, there's a new flurry of motion to his left, and pausing, he looks over once more to see the same alarming sight: His captain is again pushing up the throttles for takeoff.

Now they have the ATC clearance, but they've still not been cleared for takeoff, and yet Jacob is determined to go!

The copilot is all too aware of his dilemma. He's just corrected and embarrassed the most senior pilot at KLM and survived to tell about it. Telling Jacob a second time that he's screwing up is all but unthinkable, yet they are still not cleared to move. With the throttles coming up, the 747 will be doing just that within seconds.

Looking for a way out without further challenging or embarrassing his captain, the copilot decides to clear himself for takeoff, expecting that the tower controller will immediately order them to stay put. With his transmit button still pressed at the end of his read-back of the ATC clearance, the copilot adds a single phrase: "And...we are now at takeoff."

In the mix of languages the proper phrase in Aviation English has eluded the copilot. There is no formally approved phrase along the lines of, "We are at takeoff," but there is an approved Aviation

English phrase: "In takeoff position." For a microsecond, the tower controller lets the mental comparison of what he's heard and what he expects to hear bounce around his consciousness, and with the same propensity that most humans have to fill in the blanks and decide what someone *really* meant when there was ambiguity, he presses his button in reply.

"Okay," he says, followed by a pause of several seconds while he considers KLM's strange phraseology. Two seconds of unmodulated radio noise follows until the controller adds a single phrase: "Standby, I will call you."

At the same moment, unseen somewhere on the surface of the now foggy airport, another pilot equally unsure of what KLM means now presses his transmit button to ask for a clarification. But two transmitters trying to be heard on the same frequency at the same time only produce a loud squeal known as a heterodyne. The unseen pilot's question and the tower controller's statement cover each other, and the only sound heard in the headset of the three KLM pilots after the word "Okay" is a loud, indecipherable squeal.

The copilot needs to serve his captain's interests, and his captain wants to be cleared for takeoff immediately, and in fact thinks he already has been. So even though takeoff clearances are never issued with a single word, the copilot accepts the response and decides there is no further cause for alarm. The copilot cleared himself for takeoff, and the tower controller agreed.

In fact, in his mind, the copilot has said, "We are now pushing the power up to start rolling down the runway and accelerate to 142 knots for takeoff." However, in the mind of the controller, the KLM copilot meant: "We are in position for takeoff with the brakes on and awaiting your clearance." The total failure to understand each other under pressure was the act that pulled a trigger on a cocked and loaded gun.

"We gaan," adds Jacob in Dutch, meaning "we go."

Putting any further concerns behind him, the copilot turns all his professional attention to assisting the captain in setting the engines at the right takeoff power and watching the white center stripes jump at them faster and faster out of the fog ahead as Jacob works the nose wheel steering to keep the huge jet aligned.

20 knots. 30 knots.

Just behind the pilot's and copilot's seats in the 747's cockpit sits the flight engineer/second officer, also a qualified pilot very senior as a flight engineer and very junior to the copilot, who is very junior to the chief pilot.

40 knots.

Another radio transmission crackles through the KLM headsets, but only the flight engineer is paying attention.

"Okay, we'll report when we're clear."

To the engineer, something isn't right, and at 45 knots, completely disregarding the reality of whom he is about to interrupt and essentially question, the flight engineer leans between the seats.

"Is he not clear then, that Pan Am?"

All of them are very aware that there is another Boeing 747 in the mix of airplanes at Tenerife, and Pan Am in particular has been audibly irritated on the radio that KLM was blocking its path. Now, suddenly, the flight engineer is wondering aloud in the middle of a critical takeoff whether Pan Am is clear of the runway they're using. Aside from being a potential insult to Captain van Zanten, it essentially constitutes questioning his judgment, a fact the engineer has ignored until this moment.

50 knots.

Jacob responds with clear irritation, his concentration interrupted.

"What?"

The copilot chimes in, adopting an equally irritated tone.

"What?"

60 knots.

And the flight engineer, suddenly realizing who he has just challenged and how ridiculous it is to assume that a mere engineer could know more than the most senior and respected captain at KLM, changes his tone and focuses on trying to extricate himself from the embarrassment with a quick explanation.

"Is he not clear, that Pan Am?" The words are the same but the tone says, "Please forgive me; that was a stupid question."

"Yes!" snaps the captain.

"Yes!" echoes the copilot.

And the flight engineer slinks back into silence, undoubtedly wondering how he could have been so brazen and stupid.

80 knots.

90 knots.

100 knots.

There is still no break in the fog, and they have 42 knots to go before having enough speed to rotate the 747's nose up, letting the huge wings create lift greater than the weight it's levitating.

105 knots.

But the fog is still nothing more than clouds blowing across the surface, and suddenly they part ahead of the KLM jet, permitting a bubble of visibility as much as 3,000 feet wide.

112 knots.

The visible part of the runway contains a specter, a true nightmare. Ahead, sideways on the runway and blocking it, is the very airplane the second officer had worried about. Pan Am's 747 has missed a turn in the fog and is now blocking the runway sideways, just 1,500 feet ahead of a jumbo jet 30 knots shy of flying speed.

Jacob has nowhere to go. Too fast to swerve or stop and too slow to fly, he utters an oath and yanks the yoke back into his chest as far as it will go, his only option to leapfrog his heavily loaded jumbo over the back of the Pan Am 747, using a narrow cushion of pressurized air called ground effect — even though it's all but certain he'll climb too high too soon and crash on the other side.

For a few agonizing seconds passing in time-dilated slow motion it looks like the desperate move is going to work. The KLM 747 lifts reluctantly like a roused whale from the runway surface even as the startled Pan Am flight crew tries to jam their throttles to full power in a doomed attempt to get out of the way. Approaching like a monster from which running is impossible, the KLM jumbo closes on Pan Am, and its nose gear passes safely over the back of the Pan Am 747. But the body gear and wing landing gear of the KLM jumbo are hanging too low, and at 112 knots — almost 126 miles per hour — the galaxy of wheels and metal struts slams into and through the coach section of Pan Am, obliterating the cabin and most of its occupants. The collision rips the landing gear from the body of the KLM along with nearly 40 knots of airspeed, and the crippled plane that emerges on the other side is no longer airborne. It is ballistic and out of control, full of fuel, and mortally wounded. With agonizing certainty it descends to the runway and begins to break up, tumbling into a raging fireball and disappearing into the fog, the entire sequence unseen from the tower.

On the side of the runway and equally invisible to the tower, the burning wreckage of Pan Am's shattered fuselage separates from the wings and crumples to the ground, permitting only a handful of Pan Am's passengers, crew, and the three Pan Am pilots to escape the inferno. As a Pan Am passenger in complete shock snaps a picture of the burning wreckage, emergency crews began searching for the aircraft, unaware there are two, not one, destroyed 747's that have just come together in a version of the worst-case scenario some had predicted years earlier when 747's first took to the skies.

And within 45 seconds, 583 people are dead or dying.

Why?

If we apply the same reasoning we've always used in health care, it's obvious *someone* had to be responsible, and thus to blame, and clearly that "someone" was the captain. Rushed to depart and pushing himself and his crew, Captain Jacob van Zanten had failed to catch the fact that he was departing without a takeoff clearance, and in our traditional way of approaching such things, an error of that magnitude would simply constitute an unforgivable professional breach.

So, if he was capable of committing an unforgivable professional breach (the thinking would normally go), then Jacob van Zanten was not competent to be at the controls of that aircraft on that day in that situation, and if KLM was at fault in any way as a company and a system, it was only to the extent that it had selected the wrong man to command that flight.

But there was a huge problem with this type of traditional reasoning: Jacob was the best aviation had to offer. Regardless of how badly he'd failed and how many mistakes he'd made, he was one of those anointed mavens who were presumed by the culture to be incapable of making serious mistakes, let alone mistakes that could kill 583 people. The contradiction was all but paralytic for traditionalists and for the deeply shocked and saddened KLM family. But for the wider world of airline piloting, the accident at Tenerife, and the reality of who had triggered it, infused a deep introspection from which no one could hide: If someone like van Zanten could fail so horribly, why would there be any reason to assume that any other pilot, however senior or accomplished, would not be equally prone to another such fatal mistake?

If all pilots are subject to catastrophic mistakes as individuals, and if catastrophic mistakes are not tolerable, something had to change or air safety would never improve. Once a culture reaches such a collective catharsis of reasoning, there is no turning back.

But then there was the second part of the equation: The information that could have saved everyone aboard had been in that cockpit all along but couldn't be passed in time to the captain. In other words, aside from the basic mistake itself — beginning the takeoff without the appropriate clearances — the last, best chance for avoiding the catastrophe that followed would have been for either the copilot or flight engineer, or both, to speak up or otherwise cause the captain to stop the takeoff.

The copilot — before reaching the assumption that the tower had agreed they could takeoff — knew there was a serious problem and that the captain had forgotten not once, but twice, that he didn't have clearance to move. The flight engineer, moments later, had a snippet of information that was the last chance to avoid the start of the final accident dynamics, but he was unable to pass it along with sufficient force and lacked the authority to yank the throttles back on his own. The culture of airline piloting beat down their cautions — the culture that said that the captain must always be right, or at the very least be afforded extreme deference. That powerful cultural impetus infected all three men to the extent that even when the flight engineer spoke up, the startled captain and copilot had immediately assumed the engineer could not possibly be right and instantly dismissed his concern. Worse, realizing that he had violated the cultural dictate by questioning even for a moment his captain's judgment, the flight engineer had immediately reversed course and all but apologized for his outburst.

One of the tragic aspects of this cultural predisposition was that although Jacob was uncharacteristically grumpy that day, he never indicated either by reputation or by action that he didn't want his crew's input. His mistake, in other words, was exacerbated and perpetuated by a culture that expected individual perfection and discounted the value of operating as a crew. In fact, an extremely dangerous malady that equally infects medicine was operating in that cockpit — the halo effect, which is the tendency to believe that someone more experienced and senior could not be wrong and you be right. It is the tendency to paint a mental "halo" over the head of a respected leader, vesting in him or her capabilities of infallibility that are impossible for anyone to achieve.

Behind Every Disaster is a Tragically Flawed Assumption

There was one overriding and significant revelation from the facts of the Tenerife tragedy that essentially lay dormant and undiscussed for nearly 30 years — the role of assumption. As we've come to accept at St. Michael's, the three big error-producing tendencies of professionals are Perception, Assumption, and botched Communication. We perceive things incorrectly at critical times, we have a really hard time understanding how poorly we communicate, but when it comes to assumption, the potential for disaster is incredible, both in aviation and medicine.

Consider the copilot in Tenerife the moment he heard the tower controller speak the word, "Okay." This was a highly trained professional airman with many thousands of hours of flight experience in large jetliners, but it is a safe bet that never in his career had he ever heard a single-word takeoff clearance. Take a Boeing 747, weighing over 800,000 pounds, lined up for takeoff on a transpacific flight at Chicago (for instance), and the pilot transmits "O'Hare Tower, United eight-fifty-heavy ready to go three-two-right." The type of reply and takeoff clearance heard hour-by-hour, day-by-day at any large airport would be: "United eight-fifty-heavy, cleared for takeoff, three-two-right." But imagine in such a strict and standardized culture a controller pressing his transmit button in response and replying with a single word: "Okay." No identification of the flight, no identification of which runway, just a single term, "Okay." Never is a takeoff clearance issued anywhere in the world in the form of a single word, yet KLM's highly experienced copilot accepted just that at Tenerife. Why? Because the force and effect of the airline pilot culture and the need to serve his captain drove the copilot's desire to hear what he really wanted to hear, and anything even remotely close would have been acceptable.

What surgeon hasn't asked a question during a tense procedure and accepted the answer if it was anywhere close to what he wanted to hear? Imagine how many nurses and perfusionists and anesthesiologists have done the same thing when they knew the attending surgeon was very intent on getting on with the procedure. One of the most important things aviation has learned is that human factor mistakes increase when people are in a hurry.

This is human nature in a system that discounts human nature. But at Tenerife, it was the culture that permitted the presumption of command infallibility, and the culture that doomed them all.

Is van Zanten responsible?

If he were a doctor or a nurse, how would we feel? From medicine's perspective there is no doubt. Of *course* he was responsible, just like someone has to be responsible for a wrong-site surgery or a botched diagnosis.

But wait a minute. What does that determination do for us or for the patient, or the patient's family, if the patient doesn't survive his encounter with our system? Does fingering an individual as the responsible party in any way prevent a repeat, especially when there are many systemic elements that allowed, supported or contributed to the accident? Absolutely not. And that is another great lesson of Tenerife and a hundred other aviation accident investigations: There is never just one cause, and no such thing as a root cause, in any medical disaster or near-disaster. While the systemic element does not cancel the need for maintaining an accountable professional responsibility, future disasters from similar causes will only be prevented by addressing and fixing every single contributing factor. In other words, any contributing causal factor, if not aggressively addressed and neutralized, will more than likely become part of a dissimilar, but equally deadly, chain of causation leading to some future disaster.

In summary, after Tenerife, the old-style pecking order that led to excessive deference to a captain (and the implicit assumption that a human captain could be perfect), clearly had to be abolished. The reticence of subordinate crewmembers to stop a takeoff regardless of who was in the captain's seat had to end as well, along with any reluctance to immediately question a clearly unusual or suspect radio call. But then, too, the culture had to change to accommodate, encourage and reward subordinates for speaking up when needed.

Tenerife didn't cause overnight change in aviation's culture any more than the IOM report caused instant change in the underlying medical culture of assumed autonomy and individual perfection. But both began the process — one in 1977, ours in 1999.[3]

CHAPTER THREE

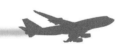

Another glass of wine had appeared on the table and Will glanced at it with no memory of its arrival. There were more pages to Jack's recitation, and he found himself compelled to read on:

Bear with me, folks, I'm not a writer. I'm a physician on a mission and even in print I'm occasionally too blunt, too hyperbolic and too enthusiastic. Please forgive bad context, mixed metaphors, periodic cheerleading, and what appear to be (and are) occasional directives as I try to impart to you why this hospital stands apart from just about all others in terms of patient safety, patient satisfaction and staff satisfaction.

By the way, if you're just coming aboard as medical staff, or considering doing so, and these new protocols and philosophies offend you or make you nervous, please go away. No kidding. We know what we're doing, we know how well it works, and while we're always very eager to learn from our new members, we will NOT put up with even the most esteemed and experienced practitioners coming in with a resistant, "This is the way I've always done it" attitude. Frankly, there are plenty of unenlightened medical centers across the state and the nation that require nothing new of you and will welcome you just as you are. We, however, have no time for, and no room for, fiercely independent practitioners who believe only they have all the answers (a description, by the way, that used to apply to me).

You see, I'm a hard-case convert, which means I understand all sides of the equation of professional resistance because I've lived it and fought change. Suffice it to say, I understand how hard change can be in these confusing times when what they told you to expect of your career seems light years away from reality. But I also know how profoundly satisfying the changes in thinking we require of you can be when you finally understand and embrace them as a better way to practice.

Frankly, no matter how much I may think of my own capabilities as a physician, I can't shrink from the reality that, thanks to the very different ways we think and act here, our patients are vastly safer. I know that some of us roll our eyes at the Hippocratic Oath as unsophisticated and idealistic, and that's sad, but here we've re-centered our dedication to the part of it that says, "*First, do no harm.*" I'm not just talking about reaffirming an ancient oath and holding hands around a campfire and singing *Kumbaya.* I'm talking about adopting a steely-eyed dedication to the belief that we can't keep our patients safe from unnecessary injury and hurt unless we practice in lockstep with the patient's best interests. And we can't do that without real mutual respect for each other, nor without true teamwork characterized by open communication and controlled egos.

You'll find something else very startling here: We all but celebrate our mistakes, because they are invaluable messages from the underlying system and often early warnings of disasters we can avoid. We openly, seamlessly and unashamedly share our failures and goofs as eagerly as we share our successes. We teach and learn from one another constantly, regardless of who has more or less experience or rank, and we change our ways of doing things by the day and sometimes the hour (yes, like Toyota). Whenever we can, we apply lessons learned and improve our methods. We have absolutely outlawed the phrase and the concept of, "This is the way we've always done it." In my view, this is the most dangerous phrase in medical practice.

Oh, and one more accolade for us: We're generally a far happier bunch than the typical hospital crew. I think you'll see some hard evidence of this as you walk through our modest "C" suite — you know, the hallway that opens onto the offices where we "CEOs" and "COOs" and "CFOs" hang out. Look at the pictures hanging there and you'll think you're at Southwest Airlines headquarters, because they're all shots of St. Michael's staff members and families having fun and celebrating together. You might say that despite the serious nature of our profession, we're deadly serious about enjoying the relationships we have with one another.

And, by the way, I think it's important to point out that we are *not* one of those institutions that view monetary success as some violation of public duty. In fact, we want our professionals to be well rewarded for their performance and the constant use of their intellect.

Want to work with people too scared of you to advise the big doc about a new procedure or tell the senior nurse about a mistake they suspect you're making? Looking forward to being with an organization that pays blind deference to your professional experience and omniscience? Do you secretly enjoy snarling at someone you consider an underling, putting them in their place, and perhaps asking sarcastically where they went to medical school? Then this isn't the place for you, and please don't let the door hit you in the rear on the way out. But, if you want to work with a good team of dedicated, energetic professionals for whom the practice of medicine centers around the patient's well being (and not our own misguided sense of medicine as an individual art), and if you are truly dedicated to using teamwork to find the best solutions, we may just be your dream job.

What We Think

First, before you can understand the basics of the radical St. Michael's philosophy, you absolutely must have a deep and humble acceptance of the reality that none of us — including me — can avoid being human and making life-threatening mistakes.

By the way, that philosophy can be stated like this: We are a group of like-minded professionals who realize that while we can't achieve perfect performance individually, we *can* achieve it as a mutually-supportive and flawlessly communicating team. We refuse to be divided by professional differences, rivalries, silos or indifference to the patient's well-being. Our common goal is the best care possible for our patients, and enjoying our careers in the process, and both parts of that equation, in that order, are our Prime Directive (an old *Star Trek* phrase).

We're going to indoctrinate you thoroughly in the three basic tiers of our highly effective patient safety and service quality system, and we're going to delve deeply into the ways that we carbon-based humans fail. But don't forget for a minute that at the center of every-thing we are at St. Michael's, and everything we've accomplished, is a universal acceptance of our own human nature. Unlike almost every other modern organization, we've let go of the dangerous ego-driven ideas we were taught in medical school, nursing school, pharmacy school, etc.

In any event, suspend disbelief and traditional thinking for a while and read on.

Why Aviation?

Many of us, if not most of us, in health care have read and heard at least something about the usefulness of the aviation industry and the nuclear power industry as models for how to improve our patient safety precautions. But in truth, too many of us have made the mistake of thinking that a business as technically precise as flying air-planes could never teach anything to the incredibly messy and complex practice of curing imprecise humans. But we naysayers, in a word, have been wrong.

Here's the bottom line: If you're to be a part of this profes-sional family and accept our common goal, you absolutely must put aside such prejudices.

Consider this truth: We in medicine have failed to put our own house in order, so we have no choice but to learn from other human endeavors.

I can't emphasize this point enough. Here we are the better part of a decade after the IOM report of 1999 (To Err is Human), and just under two decades after Dr. Lucian Leape and colleagues at Harvard validated the fact that up to 100,000 patients a year die from medical mistakes in American hospitals,[4,5] and we're still killing about the same number of patients annually. And, no, those deaths and injuries from fully preventable errors are NOT an inevitable byproduct of medical practice.

Let me put that in graphic perspective. During the same five-year period in which passenger deaths aboard major U.S. airlines hit a total of zero (2001 to 2006), American hospitals killed an esti-mated 250,000 to 500,000 patients with medical mistakes. *That's the equivalent of crashing approximately 1,400 fully loaded Boeing 747's with no survivors!*

Clearly, we still haven't learned what we need to learn to protect our patients (and ourselves), and therefore only misguided professional snobbery would prevent us from looking to other professions for guidance in what is, after all is said and done, a shared human problem.

Medical mistakes are merely human mistakes committed within a human system inadequately designed to catch and neutralize those mistakes in time.

Tenerife is about human failures, not airline failures. Tenerife is about the same halo effect that kills patients when a circulating nurse assumes a respected senior surgeon could not possibly be making the mistake she just saw. Tenerife is about the impossibility of passing important safety information in a culture that strongly discourages questioning the assumed omnipotence and infallibility of leadership. Tenerife is about the ways humans fail to communicate, fail by making deadly assumptions that are left unquestioned, and fail by perceiving things incorrectly without the assistance of a collegial team to help correct misperceptions. And Tenerife is just one of many, many examples from an industry that has killed thousands of people very publicly in order to learn an invaluable set of lessons about the reliability of inevitably flawed human institutions.

"Sir?"

Will looked up abruptly, feeling like he was swimming up from a deep REM sleep.

"Sorry?"

"I didn't mean to startle you, sir. Are you ready to order?"

There was no way to avoid yanking his wrist into view to check his watch. He'd sat down at 5:45 p.m., and now it was nearly 7 p.m.

"Good grief, I lost track of the time. Give me a second with the menu."

The waiter remained in position as Will selected a salad, then thought better of it and changed to something more substantial to fuel the impending late night watch in the ER. He'd never practiced emergency medicine as a subspecialty, but had always slightly envied those physicians who did, especially considering their airline pilot-style schedules with many days off and virtually no patient follow-ups to worry about. He couldn't imagine how St. Michael's ER could be that radically different from everyone else's version, but the people Jack Silverman had introduced in their brief foray through the ER had echoed Silverman in promising a very different experience, and he was looking forward to the details.

Showtime is 8 p.m. Enough time to eat and keep reading for awhile.

Somehow he felt roiled inside, vaguely upset and off balance, as if the story Silverman had just told was somehow threatening to him personally. But why? He'd already been familiar with the Tenerife disaster. Why would Silverman's take on it be so deeply unsettling?

The haunting image of Captain van Zanten sitting in his captain's seat and looking back at a photographer a year before he died hung in Will's mind. The picture had ended up being the key part of a two-page slick magazine ad for KLM published in dozens of magazines all over the world. In fact it was still in circulation the day the two 747s came together. Presumably, many copies of that very ad were lost in the flames that consumed Jacob and his passengers.

But it wasn't the irony or pathos of the fact that their best and brightest had been at the helm of the worst airline accident in history, Will realized. What was shaking him was how many *Doctor* van Zantens he had known throughout his career, from internship on. How many van Zantens had he worked with, worked beside, admired and even emulated? These were good people, good doctors, trained to their last breath to be perfect in every way and 10-times more brutal on themselves than anyone else would ever be for any failure. Suddenly, Will could see that they were human in a way he'd never quite envisioned.

And finally he could grasp the origin of the feeling that had been so unsettling. Seeing van Zanten as Jack's narrative presented him was like looking into a mirror, and it hit far too close to home, as if the face in that mirror — in that cockpit — was himself as CEO.

Jack Silverman was right, he thought. Van Zanten could just as easily have been a doctor or hospital CEO. And those 583 deaths — including van Zanten's — could have been a single patient fallen victim to the medically entrenched doctrine of professional infallibility.

But how on earth, Will wondered, does one even begin to hope for a change in a culture so entrenched and determined to stay unchanged and on course, however large the icebergs in its path? The enormity of the challenge melded with the image of the "van Zanten" who had been in charge the night his best friend's son had died.

CHAPTER FOUR

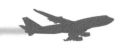

Jack Silverman took the words without comment as he moved his breakfast from the cafeteria tray to the table he'd indicated.

"You were right, of course," Will was saying. "I've never seen an ER run that way."

"You get enough sleep?"

"Not really, but that's quite all right. I got up at 5 a.m. to read the materials you provided."

Silverman finished arranging his food and picked up a fork before looking at Will.

"So, what was lesson number one?"

"Collaboration. I never saw a single decision made last night unilaterally. Everything was a consult."

"That offend you, Will?" Silverman grinned and buttered a roll, aware his younger colleague was mulling over an answer. "Yeah, I think it does."

"Well, no, but..."

"But as a physician," Jack cut in, "...there's something unsettling watching a doctor asking and not telling, right? Especially in an ER where split-second decisions are necessary?"

"Well..."

"Will, you've been a CEO and I'll wager there were plenty of times you wanted to pound the heck out of some doc who refused to conform to the house rules you wanted enforced, am I right?"

"Yeah. More than a few times."

"But you're a physician, too, so when you returned to the ranks, you realized that you now had even more power than you had as a CEO — at least in some ways."

Will was staring at his host now and nodding slowly, trying to get ahead of whatever Silverman's point might be. "I don't understand the relevance," he said at last, slightly irritated that Silverman had begun chuckling in response.

"Of course you don't. Not yet. What you saw last night among the doctors and the nurses — correct me if I'm wrong — but what you saw appeared to be weakness on the part of the physicians, and that threatens anyone with an MD who feels beaten into submission by insurance companies, lawyers and even the Joint Commission. How do we view it? Doctors who have to consult too much are unsure of themselves, and we were taught to abhor that sort of conduct or that sort of image, right? Not to mention the self-doubt."

"Yes."

"Well, my friend, what you saw was the exact opposite of weakness. What you saw were physicians who didn't feel the need to act like feral tomcats and go around marking their territory."

"Marking territory is a bit harsh as a metaphor, isn't it, Jack?"

"Absolutely not! That's not necessarily a pejorative. Every professional has that tendency, not just in health care or the physician ranks. Our position in the hierarchy is where we get our identity.[6] We're carefully trained to be the top of the medical food chain. We're taught by our medical school professors to impress that king-of-the-jungle image on anyone who might challenge our autonomy. Autonomous medical decisions become the way we practice because we're trained to be fearful of losing control, and people who are not in awe of you or scared of you might challenge your ability to issue orders with no backtalk. So, no, marking territory is as much a human trait and a trait shared by all doctors and airline captains and corporate leaders as it is the trait of the alpha wolf in a wolf pack. Even some of our female docs do exactly the same thing at times, to one degree or another."

"My point, Jack, is this," Will replied, still holding the unbitten breakfast sandwich, "I saw great collaboration, but there are times a physician has to just make a decision and move ahead. I mean, last night, the nurses and even the EMTs would approach these docs, apparently with their approval, and suggest a diagnosis or a course of treatment. It was obvious to me that they were used to getting away with that."

"And suggesting solutions and a possible diagnosis based on past professional experience is a problem, *why*?"

"Because, from a clinical point of view, it gives a physician the opportunity to jump at the first explanation and solution, and that tendency is usually a mistake, clinically speaking."

"That's entirely true. A tendency to accept the first plausible explanation is always a threat to a sound diagnosis. But let me understand your argument. You're saying that nurses and EMTs — having not been initiated in the physician's secret society — are incapable of recognizing a syndrome they've seen maybe 50 times before?"

"No, Jack, not incapable, but..."

"Here's my point. It's up to the physician to be aware that the advice given by a non-physician has to be vetted and filtered through the physician's expertise before being accepted. But we have developed the dangerous idea that a suggestion is a serious challenge to our position as doctors. Someone's invading our territory and we have to defend it against interlopers. Will, how many points of view does a physician bring to the party?"

"Well, it depends."

"Spoken like a lawyer. No, Will, it doesn't depend on anything. A physician or even a CEO or COO brings one single, solitary point of view. Yes, he's often right the first time, and he has the most education, but other points of view need to be taken into account. Ever make a bad diagnosis and had to change it later when you received more information?"

"Of course, Jack. Who hasn't?"

"Right. It's a universal experience. Wouldn't it have served the patient's best interests if you'd had that better information sooner?"

"Of course," Will replied, chewing his lip and feeling uncomfortable. Something about the exchange was really bothering him, and he couldn't decide what it was — maybe being questioned like a student, or the realization that Jack Silverman was boring into areas he'd never fully considered as a physician. Regardless, he was hovering on the horizon of irritation.

"You did read my Tenerife write-up, right?" Silverman asked, his voice a bit lower, as if sensing Will's discomfort.

"Yes. It was terrifying and very enlightening. I also read your — what did you call it — introduction to 'us.' And, frankly, it was a bit harsh."

"Let me ask you this, Will. And I have a solid reason for the inquisition here, aside from the fact I like the Socratic method of teaching. How many professional points of view did the captain have in that cockpit before pushing the power up?"

"One, of course. His guys couldn't speak to him because of the culture."

"Right, and the culture reinforced that. It even infected the copilot and the flight engineer, who at various times beat back their own independence of thought — their own ability to form an opinion of what was real and safe and what wasn't — in favor of conforming not just to the captain's view of the world, but to the point of view that there was only one competent arbiter of whether it was safe to go. We do the same thing when a physician resents in any way, openly or covertly, the fact that someone without an MD offered an idea, an opinion, or horror-of-horrors, a diagnosis without having the secret handshake."

"I still say we do have to be careful about accepting the first idea that comes along."

"Granted, and that's where professional responsibility comes in. We have to be Jean-Luc Picard."

"Ah... excuse me?"

"*Star Trek* reference. I'll explain later. There's so much to tell you. You're probably sensing already that the way I'm approaching these traditionally held views might be uncomfortable."

"Unfamiliar, Jack, not necessarily uncomfortable."

"Fair enough. Look, let me give you an extreme example of what I call the John Wayne Defense of professional autonomy."

"You do like pop culture references, don't you, Jack?"

"I certainly do. They're shared experiences — movies and TV shows. I use them because the mere mention of a title or a scene can often instantly align two individuals' understanding of something. The John Wayne Defense, in other words, is about circling the wagons."

"An aggressive reaction."

"Aggressive, knee-jerk, single-minded and absolutely righteous. No need to reexamine anything. Circle them wagons against the barbarians who are not doctors."

"Okay."

"Or, Will, the 'C' suite tendency to circle the wagons against those who are not corporate officers."

"I'm getting it."

"About a year ago we brought a talented orthopod in here who we now know got his privileges under false pretenses. I did the screening and gave him a thumbs-up because he said all the right things, but when he got into routine practice and started sending patients to the nurses in the orthopedics wing, his true nature came out almost immediately. Problem for him, he didn't realize he was walking into a transparent culture totally different from anything he'd experienced. He thought he had a covey of victims at his disposal, and he set about training them in his fashion. Now, this guy was anything but the typical physician. In fact, he represents perhaps a maximum of 5 percent of the entirety of physicians. But let me tell you, Will. Never minimize how just one bad apple can spoil the whole communication culture. Turns out the man was angry at the world, newly divorced, making far less than he'd been told to expect as a doctor, and if he had a screw loose it was in the direction of being a bit sadistic. In his previous hospitals he'd been getting by with unreported abusive conduct toward staff for years because the nurses and even the hospitalists around him were too afraid of the man's withering disdain to challenge him, let alone risk turning him in. But here at St. Michael's, it took all of two days for our nurses to sound the alarm and let us know in no uncertain terms that we'd mistakenly given privileges to a Mr. Hyde masquerading as Dr. Jekyll. Moreover, because they were sure of our support, they calmly collected the objective proof we needed."

"What, they caught the guy on camera or on tape?"

"The nurses didn't have to. All they needed was two or more of them, because they know we trust them. No, what they did was carefully document, almost chart, this man's abusive forays onto the floor and the OR. I called a meeting with the staff on the third day to review those reports. This guy, who'd pretended to be so enthralled with our unique methods, had come charging into the unit purposefully snarling at, belittling, and intimidating everyone, ordering the nurses and even the nurse-manager to memorize his variations on post-op procedures with everything from steri-strips to turning patients. He was insulting, intimidating, disdainful and just plain disrespectful. Now, Will, the sad part is that act would have worked for him in most hospitals, but our gals and guys were totally unintimidated because they knew they had full support all the way to the top. They tried to address the behavior by themselves, and when that didn't work, three of them coordinated a written account. By day four — no kidding, just day four — this surgeon thought he had his territory fully marked and that everyone was shaking in their boots and ready to obey him without question. A Marine boot camp drill instructor wouldn't have used a different approach."

"So how did you handle him? When I was CEO, I would have had a devil of a time just getting rid of him."

"I had one of our longtime orthopods ask the man to lunch on day four to draw him out. Dr. Bill Munori. But the lunch just turned out to be a confirmation and even an embellishment of the information we had already gathered from staff.

Turns out, this abusive guy had spent eight years in a very large, very well-known hospital in Houston, and he told Bill that he was so angry at nurses for having the audacity to make suggestions about medications and challenging his expertise that he routinely spent his evenings scouring the pharmaceutical literature so he could maintain a list of alternative medications for the times a nurse would have the temerity — as he put it — to call and recommend a course of action.[7] He would, he said, immediately counter that she was recommending something that could kill the patient, scare her into thinking she was about to make a hideous mistake, and then order the other medication, whether it was the best choice or not. He was, he said, determined to do his part to stamp out that type of arrogance on the part of non-physicians, and if a patient suffered a little in the process, it was for a good cause. Word for word, Will."

"I take it he no longer has privileges?"

"We aligned our medical staff and hospital board bylaws, and

I have the power to eliminate a bad apple. I called him in the next day, took his badge, told him why, and had security march him to the door. Can you imagine the look on this guy's face? Now, maybe that's marking *my* territory, but I went immediately to the floor he'd tried to terrorize, called a meeting of as many staff as I could find, and told them precisely what I'd done and why."

"I'll bet they were overjoyed."

"No, in fact they felt sorry for the guy, that he was so twisted around and incapable of thinking of them as teammates and colleagues. Will, they had full confidence that I would do exactly what I did, without hesitation. We're a family, and this guy couldn't understand the first thing about collaboration, let alone mutually supportive, nurturing relationships. As a matter of fact, there are several hard-hitting studies out now that validate the damage disruptive behavior can have on everything from nurse satisfaction and retention, to the actual outcomes of patient care. And that's whether it's a nurse or a physician who's being disruptive. We cannot tolerate it in health care any longer.[8,9] By the way, there's an excellent book out called *Ending Nurse-to-Nurse Hostility: Why Nurses Eat Their Young and Each Other*, which should be required reading for every member of every health-care 'C' suite, especially those who think things are going swimmingly well in the nurse department. Nurses are in crisis, and with a low professional self-esteem and a national paradigm of discounted worth, inadequate staffing and senior nursing leaders typically far too disconnected and powerless to change things, nurses act like rats in an overcrowded cage and turn on one another."[10]

Will had been munching the breakfast sandwich, deep in thought, as Silverman talked. He washed down the last of it with coffee and realized Jack Silverman was waiting for a response.

"I've seen that kind of nurse-against-nurse attack, but I didn't know it was endemic. I've also known guys like your problem-child orthopod," Will began, "and you're right — it's really hard to catch them in the act."

Silverman was shifting in his chair, as if getting a new physical grip on the surroundings before resuming his command of the subject.

"It's the bell curve, Will."

"I... understand bell curves, of course, but how are you applying it?"

"Like this. Our renegade orthopod, as I said, represents a tiny 5 percent of the force of physicians. He's on the extreme end — the bad end — of the physician bell curve. On his end, there's no collaboration, no teamwork, and nothing but a single point of view rendered in an environment of hate, hostility and defensiveness, often to cover up massive insecurity. Making a suggestion, however innocent or well-intentioned, is seen as an attack. But where's the middle of the curve, Will?"

"That would be where you and I and most docs would practice. Good practitioners who interact well with the staff and care about the patients while maintaining objectivity. Right?"

Silverman was nodding as he sat back. "We always thought that way, didn't we? Obviously, you still do, and you've run a hospital."

"So I have it wrong?"

"Not wrong, Will. You have an incomplete picture. See, the middle of the bell curve is in the wrong place, because too many physicians under its down slope — the one leading in the direction of the minority that orthopod represented — feel much like he did, but they're far more subtle. They don't snarl at nurses, they just don't say anything. They don't belittle directly, they just refuse to learn the first names of people they've worked with for years. They don't openly discount or ignore a nurse's observation or opinion on the floor or the ER or the ICU. They just make nurses feel inferior by never asking for their opinions or bothering to read the nursing notes in the chart. Or they snap a little when they have to answer a page, and sometimes unload on the nurse who is injudicious enough to have a patient in severe pain without orders at 3 a.m. Nurses, Will. Our eyes and ears on the front lines where our patients are struggling to recover! They achieve the same alienation of their non-physician colleagues by simply denying their relevancy in so many different ways, and by refusing to even acknowledge the professionals around them as fellow human beings. One of the first steps is shifting that bell curve in the right direction. That means getting everyone who has formerly felt threatened by the concept of collaboration to make the massive cultural changes needed, and to stop worrying about defending the status of MD against everyone else. It's about relaxing and working for the common goal. And it's far easier to say than to achieve."

"Jack, forgive me, but you're describing a sort of utopia."

"Which would mean an unachievable ideal. Not true. When you shift that bell curve significantly, you don't just get rid of that rancid 5 percent, but you point everyone toward empathy and cooperation and make outcasts of those who would live on the down slope toward non-collaboration. The norm must be collegiality and dependence on one another, regardless of who has what degrees. I'm harping here on physicians because you and I are physicians, and because physicians have to understand, embrace, and lead all of these changes to make them effective. Physicians simply have the power — and therefore the responsibility. The truth is, it's the covert or absent behaviors that kill teamwork by silencing communication, and thereby making it impossible to have a common goal. It's the covert or absent behaviors that keep patients in the crosshairs of human error.[11] The stuff that's never reported — the little subtle things that hurt and destroy morale and professional self esteem, and lead to hostility, hopelessness, and abandoned or apathetic careers. This is one of the major keys to patient safety, Will, and it's why medicine has made so little progress in nine years. We never realized what was causing the lack of cooperation, so we couldn't even begin to address it. All the Joint Commission or IHI or AHRQ initiatives imaginable will fall flat until physicians realize that they can no longer practice in an autonomous, aloof, and disconnected way. But, unfortunately, this is how we've been taught. The key to safety, and quality, is having people care about one another as they combine as a team for the best interests of their patients. Without that major cultural change, our efforts would be hopeless."

"Jack, did the airlines achieve that?"

"In some ways, yes. In some aspects, they only lit the way.

But what they and the nuclear power industry *have* achieved is to make it very, very clear that when it involves safety and protection from human error, an individual, no matter how professional and experienced, can never be anywhere near as reliable as a group can be. They've also given us tragic evidence that a group divided against itself by professional jealousy, stratification, or just inability to communicate, is doomed to fail. See, Will, these are things they don't tell you in those gee-whiz-here's-how-pilots-would-run-an-OR courses. But if you get people to respect and interact respectfully with one another for the common goal of helping the patient, the culture can and will change. Fail to do that, and you can bring in all the tactical methodologies you want, and in the end they'll amount to nothing."

"And the patient injury and death rate will stay the same."

"Absolutely. I'm sure you've heard the adage that, 'Culture kills the best of strategies.' Team members who feel poorly regarded by the leader are going to have the human propensity to remain disconnected from the leader and the common goal. In an extreme situation, an angry subordinate team member may actually stand back and say nothing when the leader is making a mistake just to let him prove his vulnerability by default, even if it harms a patient! Bottom line, if there's no collegiality, no mutual respect, there's no teamwork and no improvement."

"Which is why I failed," Will said, somewhat under his breath, but with enough volume that Jack Silverman nodded with his most sympathetic face. Dr. Jenkins, he could see, was getting it.

Will's Notes:

1. The willingness to assume that a suggestion from a non-MD is automatically a threat to practice autonomy is a dangerous idea. The concept of practice autonomy itself may not be a good thing, especially from a patient safety point of view.

2. Aligning the corporate bylaws of a hospital with the bylaws of the medical staff may be the key to having clear authority to enforce standards and best practices.

3. Physicians can do almost as much damage to nursing morale by not speaking or interacting with them as they can by yelling or being disruptive! I doubt a tenth of the physicians in the United States have ever considered this. These are called "covert" or "absent" behaviors.

4. Great quote: "Culture kills the best of strategies."

5. True teamwork depends on collegiality and mutual respect. And patient safety in turn depends, to an inordinate extent, on teamwork.

CHAPTER FIVE

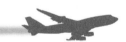

Back in Jack Silverman's office, Will shook his head as he plopped down in the offered chair across from the CEO's desk.

"Jack, if you were teaching this as a seminar for CEUs, you'd have a list of objectives, and I may need something like that to keep these ideas organized."

"I already have them written down, but let me give you the points verbally. I find people remember things better if they have to write them down."

"Okay," Will said, scrambling to poise a pen over his legal pad.

"First," Silverman began, "let me say I view the way we state formal objectives for CEUs with the same disdain I reserve for the way they ask questions on that game show, *Jeopardy!* So let me state these as lessons, not objectives. The *Prime Lesson* — I won't even number this one — is that humans will always make mistakes regardless of their training, experience or determination. In other words, the universal constant is that human infallibility is impossible, and those who build a system that depends on an absence of serious human mistakes will fail utterly."

"Okay, I couldn't agree more."

"Now, what I'll call 'Lesson Number One' is this: Since human infallibility is impossible, the only chance to keep human errors from hurting patients is by creating collegial interactive teams whose members, operating together, can catch and neutralize one another's mistakes.

"Lesson Two: Collegial interactive teams cannot be effective without mutual human caring and support.

"Lesson Three: Collegial interactive teams can never be effective unless all members of the team achieve barrierless communication, which means the ability to pass information in any direction to any member without hesitation when important information needs to be passed, and for all other purposes in the patient's best interests. And that also means the ability for any member to question any other member about anything relevant to the task without that question being taken as an insult.

"Lesson Four: Collegial interactive teams can never achieve barrierless communication if the culture allows leaders to regard ideas, suggestions, proffered opinions and even diagnoses as a challenge to the leader's authority or professional ability.

"Lesson Five: Even when a team leader is properly receptive, a team can never achieve barrierless communication if the surrounding culture successfully discourages subordinates from speaking up.

"Lesson Six: A leader whose control of his or her team is based on hierarchical snobbery and defensiveness — or whose methods of control include fear, intimidation, ignorance or superiority — can never achieve barrierless communication. Such leaders, by their actions, elicit emotional reactions that are universally counterproductive and dangerous to the interests of improved patient safety and practice quality. Hierarchical snobbery and distance, by definition, damages or destroys collegiality, self-esteem, and communication, yet most of us are abysmally unaware of how the traditional medical culture perpetuates, allows and even encourages it."

Jack Silverman waited for Will to catch up and look up.

"Okay," Will said. "Basically, Jack, you're saying that it's not just a matter of the leader telling everyone to speak up, he's got to create an environment that encourages unfettered information transfer and one that doesn't tolerate people remaining silent."

"That's the basis of what aviation did so well in the cockpit, but that's only part of the equation. Mutual caring and support on a human basis — what I characterized as Lesson Two — is also vital. What we've discovered is that it's not just a formula but an attitude — not left brain, but right brain — and you don't achieve that mutually supportive attitude without mutual professional and personal respect, which is, in turn, impossible if the leader is superior, crass, manipulative, defensive or just doesn't care about his colleagues."

"Or doesn't even consider them colleagues, as I'm afraid too many of us physicians signal unknowingly to the nurses we encounter. They're there, they're important, but..."

"Right," Jack interrupted, "but they're marginally trained subordinates supposed to be at our beck and call, and they're always supposed to be respectful if not in awe of us, as well as selfless — a job description that is a combination of martyr and mother."

"Which is the attitude we picked up in med school."

"Yep. The 'norms and mores' of the medical culture. The med school and nursing curriculums are other highly dysfunctional areas that have to be massively changed. Physician-nurse communication, or the utter lack of it in too many instances, arises from an absence of collegiality, and it's killed uncounted thousands of patients. No, probably hundreds of thousands. What we've done about that here will probably shock you more than the constant consultative atmosphere you observed in the ER last night."

"How are you defining collegiality, Jack?"

"Okay, take this example with made-up names. Dr. Jim Black and Nurse Jane Brown have been working around each other for 15 years. To him she's 'Nurse.' He's never learned or bothered to care about learning her first name, her last name, or anything about her personally. He's not a mean-spirited guy, but the physician culture has taught him that nurses are just kind of 'there,' and he's not supposed to get to know them personally. Now, this is actually a serious dichotomy. If you ask *him*, he'll tell you that it's wrong to say he was taught nurses are just there. He'll tell you he was taught that nurses are very important members of the team, and that, indeed, is the book answer in med school. But in practice — as with many human institutions — he's been taught something entirely different. In fact, the MD culture on the front lines has passed down a code of standoffish behaviors that reflect the attitude that cooperating collegially with nurses is somehow a diminishment of a physician's autonomy and power. Yet in this case and for 15 years Dr. Black has depended on that particular nurse, among others. Now, to Nurse Brown, Dr. Jim Black is always addressed as 'Doctor,' or 'Dr. Black.' She knows his first name very well, she knows where he lives, much of his background and even where he went to med school. But they've never once had a sustained personal conversation, and in her experience that just isn't expected unless the physician initiates it. There's no conflict, it's just business as usual and impersonal. They collaborate very well. But they're not really colleagues. Then one day they see each other at their kids' soccer game. Each has a kid on the same team. They start talking, and within a few games seeing each other sparks a 'Hi, Jane,' and a, 'Call me Jim.' They find they've got a lot in common, and on that neutral ground, and in that casual, human atmosphere, they end up exchanging enough personal information about each other's lives that everything changes. Suddenly she becomes human to him, a woman with a name, and he becomes a more sympathetic and real individual to her. And guess what? The next time Dr. Black hits her floor at Our Lady of Pretty Good Outcomes Hospital, they're now on a first-name basis and have at least soccer and kids in common. Professionally, they have the patient's best interests in common and can talk about disagreements with that in mind. Jane no longer hesitates to respectfully bring up concerns. And since Jane is no longer just a nameless nurse, he's automatically more considerate of her professional input. That's collegiality. What they had before was professional collaboration, but collegiality is an order of magnitude above collaboration in terms of the ability to communicate, because it's based on mutual respect and understanding and caring, however rudimentary. It enables barrierless communication as surely as an on/off switch. Equal respect begets equal power, and when you want all members of the team to be guardians of the patient, that's vital. There's no one-upmanship, and no need for either of them to raise shields against the other professionally."

"I'd never thought of that. So, if I'm understanding you, in order to achieve collegiality, you require all your people to have kids on the soccer team?" Will grinned.

"Will, if I thought that question was really serious I'd throw you out of here," Jack laughed in response, leaning forward suddenly, pointing to the legal pad. "Hey, before I continue, let me see what you wrote."

"You mean, the lessons? On this legal pad?"

"Yes."

Will handed it over somewhat reluctantly, feeling a bit like a schoolboy turning in an assignment he didn't know was now due, and Silverman took the pad and scanned the entries.

> **Prime Lesson: Humans will always make mistakes regardless of their training, experience or determination. In other words, the universal constant is that human infallibility is impossible.**
>
> 1. Since human infallibility is impossible, the only chance to keep human errors from hurting patients is by creating collegial interactive teams.
>
> 2. Collegial Interactive Teams (CIT's) cannot be effective without mutual caring and support.
>
> 3. CIT's can't be effective unless all members of the team achieve <u>Barrierless Communication (BC)</u>.
>
> 4. <u>No BC</u> if the team culture allows leaders to regard ideas, suggestions, proffered opinions and even diagnoses as an unacceptable challenge to the leader's authority or ability.
>
> 5. <u>No BC</u> if the culture successfully discourages subordinates from speaking up, regardless of the reason.
>
> 6. <u>No BC</u> if the team leader's control is based on hierarchical snobbery, defensiveness, etc. i.e., where did YOU go to med school?

Jack handed it back. "You got it, although I try to refrain from reducing everything to an acronym. We deal with too many of them as it is."

"Okay, so what do I put down for Lesson Seven?"

"Nothing until later. What I want you to do now is tell me

what else surprised you last night. What else really stood out as very different from every other ER you've experienced?"

Will sat in thought for only a few seconds before leaning forward. "Well, this was a shocker for me. One of the physicians orders IV morphine for one of the patients before he goes on a break, comes back and finds that Dilaudid has been substituted instead. I thought he was just going to change it and do what we do so often, just say nothing, or maybe he'd be one of those few on the far end of the bell curve who thinks he needs to chew out the nurse. Neither he nor I understood why the change had been made, or whether it was a mistake. But instead of reacting, he goes to the nurses' station and flips through the chart, then he looks up and actually apologizes to the nurse and thanks her for catching the fact that his patient was allergic to morphine! I was pretty sure I'd heard him wrong at first, because I looked at the chart as well and hadn't seen any warnings about allergies. But he told her it was one of those system errors they talk about, and said his contribution had apparently been in failing to realize the chart wasn't assembled before he left, which was, he said, the prime contributing cause to missing the allergy sticker.

"I can't say I was stunned, Jack, because many of us can be analytical about our mistakes. But it was his tone of voice — he said it with such an utter ease and disregard for blame and respect for the team element that it was close to surreal, and the way the nurse reacted was the same. No fear that she was going to be pounced on, no 'I told you so' attitude or smugness. She simply fell into lockstep in a joint effort to figure out why it had happened, as if it had been a major near-miss. She explained that her procedures had contributed as well because she hadn't picked up the order until after he'd left the floor. She'd had to go to the covering physician to get an order to substitute Dilaudid instead. And then there was the reinforcement. A little while later this same physician passed the same nurse in the hall, smiled, waved, and said 'Great save back there, Aggie!' with a smile and a big thumbs up. You should have seen her beam! That one act I'm sure guaranteed that she'll keep up that level of scrutiny in the future, because he made her feel good about it. I guess I never really had the distance to see it from this angle. As a physician, I was too immersed in the role, and as a CEO I was too far away to notice."

"What else?"

"Then, what really amazed me was that at the end of their shift he called a meeting of every staff member, and they huddled for 10 minutes to craft several changes in the way they handle routine pain med orders. First, they took the sequence apart like some sort of accident investigation with an ease that was really incredible, like they'd done this a thousand times before. I don't remember all the contributing factors or the timing, but essentially there should have been a red sticker on the outside of the chart placed there by the secretary. But the secretary was still assembling the chart when the doc picked up the parts of it he needed, wrote his order, and left without seeing the sticker, which was upside down on the desk. The nurse caught it because you apparently have a critical review policy for any medication."

Jack was nodding. "We have a built-in rule that says we must expect literally every medication order to contain a potentially lethal mistake. In effect, we put the burden of proof on whoever is dealing with a medication order at any point in the process to confirm that it's really correct, and the best way to confirm is having a colleague independently verify. But the built-in protective bias that works is when we truly expect without variance that the order is wrong until proven right."

"Really? You have an institutional expectation of failure?"

"Every single time."

"Well, it apparently worked, because she caught the allergy. Anyway, in this meeting, they came up with a revised primary procedure for the future in which no med order is complete for the doc until he does what is effectively a verbal handoff to the nurse with the chart in front of them. They then posted it as part of their unit procedures, and went home, just like that. They seemed to actually enjoy the process."

"And how is this unusual?"

"Jack, let me count the ways. I mean, I know you're baiting me, but first, the physician was extraordinarily honest and open about what could have been a very serious mistake."

51

"Not here. What he did was not extraordinary here, it's business as usual."

"Okay, well, it would be extraordinary everywhere else. But then there's the fact that no one was running around looking for someone to blame."

"That's because we killed the blame culture here. Stated more properly, we outlawed it and retrained all of us. I'll explain more about that later. What else?"

"Well, then there's this corrective collaborative meeting at the end of a very intense shift, and a brand new procedure drafted and actually posted in the unit procedures. I mean, people voluntarily stayed around to do this! No gun to their heads, no pending investigation, no injured patient who might sue and no Joint Commission visit imminent. They just figured it out, came up with a fix, and posted it without a medical committee review or even a signoff by the director of the ER. Just wham! Done."

"And I know I sound like a broken record, Will, but this is a problem, how?"

"No, no, no! It's not a problem, it's breathtaking. They didn't seem the slightest bit concerned that they were donating their time, looking way beyond themselves, and bypassing maybe five tiers of higher authority. In my hospital, there was an endless stream of people bringing me problems. Suggested solutions were rare, bureaucratic and took an endless number of meetings for consensus or implementation to occur."

"*Our* front lines have full authority to make changes concurrent with their immense responsibilities. When the team makes a decision, upper management had better have an overwhelmingly good reason for reviewing it, let alone trying to reverse it by fiat. In fact, we don't allow management changes by fiat, except for dire emergencies. If the director of the ER doesn't like a change, she asks the folks who made that change to come together again and take a second look at it. They don't take that as a challenge, but as a suggestion to refine things. You'd be surprised how proud a team gets when the second time around they come to the very same conclusion, knowing the ER director will fully support them. They live for unanimity. And unless what they want to do is a major and clear conflict with best practices or some external regulation or law, that's the way we're going to be doing it."

"Okay, and one final thing. I was flabbergasted at how thoroughly the nurses, including Mary, the charge nurse..."

"Glad to hear you using first names."

"Yeah, everyone does down there, but I was amazed at how well they kept the patients and family informed, and how solicitous they were of the families and friends. One fellow needed an X-ray that seemed to be taking too long and I saw Mary pop in his alcove about every five minutes to report on the progress. No bull, either. She was telling the truth about trying to chase down the radtech and the workload that had suddenly peaked. By the way, I went out and watched the admissions process as well, and even though you've conformed to the no-waiting model, it's still quite different. No flint-hard attitude, no lost patients suffering alone and forgotten in the room they were hustled into. And even when an exasperating woman was cursing up a storm at being asked ER admitting questions about her child, who was already being wheeled in, your folks were humane, courteous and very attentive."

Jack was nodding. "And you wouldn't believe how many we've had to hire and fire to get the right mix of temperaments and skill in place there. Takes empathy, Will, and a lot of it. But, clinically, there's solid reason to pay a lot of attention to — and show a lot of respect to — the people who do that job. If they don't get it right on triage, we waste time, money, talent, and create greater hazards for the patients and the hospital. We don't consider them gatekeepers, by the way. We consider them mentors, helping our patients get the right care as quickly as possible."

"Bottom line, Jack, you were right when you told me that it was amazingly different. And that's just the ER."

"You mind if we go over the 'why' again?"

"Not at all. But I didn't expect you to spend *this* much time with me."

"I get very passionate in spite of my schedule, Will, and I appreciate the fact that you're listening carefully." Jack hesitated for a second, wondering whether to press Will for any additional hints of what trauma had driven him here.

Later, he concluded.

"Okay, first, Will, what you saw last night with that interaction regarding the pain meds goes to the heart of what makes St. Michael's so different. From your own description, you could see they never lost sight of the common goal of serving the patient's best interests, and they were not defensive about discussing ways to get to that common destination with better efficiency and safety. In other words, we're not invested in the process, we're invested in the outcome. Think of it this way: The process is infinitely changeable, but the desired outcome is singular and perpetual."

"Okay, professor, but how do you get rid of the professional territoriality that usually keeps people so apart? I mean, I understand now your point that what I saw in the ER last night was cooperation, not weakness. But in order for strong physicians to practice the way they were — to interact that freely — takes a suspension of our normal concern about defending our right to make our own clinical decisions."

"First, everyone has to agree to be governed by a single process, as a single body. This is a difficult balance, Will, as you know, in any American hospital, and especially when hospitals operate more like a farmer's market than a unified enterprise. I see your eyebrows popping up. What I mean by farmer's market is just this: Most hospitals provide the roof and the tables, but the doctors, in effect, rent space to ply their trade. We all know that most physicians don't work directly for the hospital, and in at least one state, they can't even be directly employed by a hospital, which begs sanity. Yet, how can we provide the best care if everyone is off doing their own thing, arguing among themselves about which best practice data is correct or relevant to their practice, and maybe complying with clearly evident best practices and maybe not?"

Will interrupted. "I tried to recruit the best and the brightest, and what I found out was that the 'best and brightest' revered their own practices as superior to anyone else's."

"Exactly!" Jack said. "What other enterprise in this nation with such high responsibility and potential liability would tolerate the level of individual practice variation that has become standard in medicine? Try this: Would you fly on an airline that let their captains decide individually whether to use flaps or checklists, or turn on all the engines for takeoff?"

Will was shaking his head. "Of course not."

"Would you want your neighborhood nuclear power plant run in freeform, avant-garde style by a manager who thinks he's smarter than the rules and is intent on experimenting with, say, the cooling valve positions and fuel rod extraction procedures?"

"Got the point, Jack."

"Well, that's the nutty level of autonomy we permit in the average hospital, and let's call it what it is: Insanity. If I'm under the knife as a patient, I want to trust the surgeon's skill and discretion *and* the fact that he or she is going to employ the best distillation of the best practices. In other words, I want the benefit of what we've found works best, nationwide, even worldwide. Otherwise, I'm a guinea pig in an unnecessary experiment held long after the truth of what works best has been discovered. And even though I want that doc to use his or her best cognitive skills — that impossible-to-define skill that approaches art — the setup for a well-understood surgical procedure, for example, should be standardized. We don't need to reinvent the wheel with each procedure."

"How do you mean?"

"Take airplanes. We know a Boeing jetliner takes off best with some flaps extended. I'm not a pilot, but I've studied the subject. If we know that using some flap extension for takeoff is the best and safest method, why on earth would we tolerate variations? Yet, day-after-day in the vast majority of American hospitals, we ignore the fact that with many, if not most procedures, there exist well-understood and well-established best practices — established ways of doing things that work consistently and get the best patient outcomes. Not just in surgery, by the way, but equally in the ICUs, with orthopedics, with the medication process — darn near everything. Yet we say: 'Hey, do your own thing. Best practices be danged.'"

"I'll admit it seems insane. I never looked at it that way."

"We're not trained to look at it that way. It's the professional

inertia, Will. The way we've always done it, and it's cultural sui-
cide. Worse, the malpractice lawyers know what the best practices
are, and they're ready to crucify anyone who refuses to use them,
and hospitals that refuse to force the issue with their medical
staffs. And then there's the public backlash factor."

"Meaning?"

"Will, mark my words. If the American public ever catches
on — if they ever fully realize before we get it under control, the
true nature of this uncontrolled, freeform system of chaotic,
maverick practice we've perpetuated — we physicians will lose
what autonomy we have in a major firestorm of public indigna-
tion that will propel badly designed federal legislation that none
of us will be able to live with. Guaranteed."

"You really think it could come to that?"

"You have any faith in the collective intellect and balance of
the House and the Senate?"

"No more than Will Rogers had, especially not today when
they spend most of their energy trying to vanquish the opposing
party."

"Exactly. Well, they're the loony laymen who will dictate our
fate if we don't change the system in time. We recognized that
here at St. Michael's and finally admitted to ourselves that our
system made no sense. So we changed it."

"So, now you directly employ your physicians?"

"No, but we are directly engaged in the same vision. We're
as unified as if they were receiving an annual W-2. We could have
gone either way — require full employment for every physician,
or do what we did. What we've elected to do, at least in the
short-term, is massively alter our bylaws and harmonize them so
that regardless of what group the physicians' paychecks come
from, in order to practice here, they have to agree to be under
the unified practice control of this hospital. That's a specific concept, Will — unified practice control. Now, in return, we provide
exemplary transparency and constant, mainstream physician
participation in governance so no one feels dictated to by the
uninitiated. But if we establish a policy together, that policy is
not subject to the whims of an individual doctor determined to
prove he has an inherent professional birthright to practice any

way he wants to. And if we dismiss a misbehaving practitioner from privileges — like that orthopod I told you about — he or she stays dismissed. We do what we say we're going to do."

"Whoa, wait a minute! With all due respect to the fact that you're a fellow physician, Jack, doctors are just not going to agree to be under the administrative control of the hospital, when most hospitals are run by well-meaning administrators who — sorry, Jack — haven't a clue what happens on the floors."

"Absolutely right," Jack said, smiling and waiting as Will stared at him uncomprehending.

"I'm… *right*? But… I'm not following this."

"That's because you're thinking inside the box and making a typical assumption. I said 'administrative control.' That sounds to you like the despised threat of non-doctors dictating to doctors. But that's neither what I actually said, nor what we're doing."

Will's hands were up and spread open as he shook his head with a smile. "You've lost me now for sure."

"Our physicians make the medical rules, and once made, they are enforced unilaterally. But it's not administrators doing the oversight and enforcing, it's the medical staff. Unified practice control means that we achieve agreement, however painful, on what the best standards of practice are, and then apply those standards to every practitioner as if he or she was a W-2 employee."

"Oh. Isn't it that way at most hospitals?"

"No, Will. At most hospitals — probably including the one you ran — there is constant dynamic tension between and among the standards the administrator wants followed, what the standards should be in the eyes of the chief of medicine and his or her lieutenants, and the physicians, most of whom are not directly employed by the hospital and consider themselves and their various groups autonomous. That's the true model for herding tomcats. What we do is challenge our physicians to get unified on each position, and then we make sure the resulting standards are imposed firmly. They're always open to alteration, but not to exception."

"And if one of the groups doesn't want to go along with what everyone else decides?"

"We have a binding arbitration procedure for resolving medical issues over best practices and evidence-based advances, if our docs can't agree. But we've used it only twice so far. You can see, can't you, how irresponsible it is to permit a wild array of different practices when we do have the ability to figure out at least in some important cases what's best? If *we* can't figure it out, I promise the medical malpractice lawyers understand it, and that's one of the first questions being asked in depositions today: What is your practice standard for the procedure that went wrong, and if you didn't have one, why not?"

"Okay, I get it. But you're telling me that the medical staff really got behind this... unanimity?"

"Considering they were the ones who helped create it as a team, and they were the ones who argued it out and agreed to and wrote all the procedures we enforce, you bet. Was it a tumultuous time? Absolutely! Is everyone happy with every decision? Of course not. Many want direct employment, and we may do that later. Are all our procedures and standards open to continuous revision? You bet. So while we all adhere to the same practice standards wherever we've set them, those standards are a living, breathing set of procedures and rules and objectives. We'll change them several times a day if better evidence comes to light. But mavericks are not welcome here. And, in fact, you risk the professional insurance coverage we provide if you knowingly refuse to comply."

"But, Jack, when you say evidence-based..."

"I know, I know. There are a thousand areas where there is no clear evidence of what's best, especially in diagnostics, and also disparaging views on best practice, right? Was that what you were going to point out?"

"Absolutely. Otherwise we're practicing cookbook medicine."

"Which is the phrase too often used to just automatically reject evidence-based procedures and variability-reducing methods. No, Will, where real evidence exists and we can get a consensus, we adopt a policy. Where it doesn't, we leave it up to the cognitive and analytical brilliance of our docs. But this is the point! If you were a journalist from *Newsweek* or ABC with a camera crew, this would be one of the main points I'd be desperate to get across: There really is a happy and safe middle ground between cookbook medicine and a profession of uncontrolled maverick practice and, by George, we've found it! If we institute a procedure or method to improve patient safety from which no one is allowed to deviate, I don't have to enforce it from the head shed. Peer pressure alone keeps people in line. You're just not going to have the respect of your peers if you try to play the maverick card here, and people have found it's much more fun being part of a proud team."

Will saw Jack looking at his watch.

"I'm taking too much of your morning."

"No, really, I'm enjoying the back and forth here, and especially the fact that you're reporting exactly what I'd hoped you'd see last evening. But I'm going to park you in the ICU for a few hours, and then, after lunch, get you into at least one surgical procedure under the wing of our chief of surgery, Dr. Alice Quinn. You think *I'm* a vociferous advocate, wait 'til she gets through proselytizing you!"

"I can't wait, but can I get one more subject covered first?"

"Sure."

"You said in that introductory piece you give to incoming staff that there were three tiers of a safety system, and you mentioned them rather rapidly."

"Right. Those three tiers are perception, assumption and communication. To organize your thinking, look first at the subject of human fallibility. Once we agree that even the best of us make mistakes, the next question should be *how* do we fail? What are the *mechanisms* of human mistakes? That's where the big three come in — communication, assumption and perception. Most medical errors and associated human mistakes arise from miscommunication, disastrous assumptions and misperceptions."

"Misperceptions of, what — the patient?"

"Misperception of anything, Will. We humans misperceive things all the time. Ever read a clock or a watch wrong?"

"Of course."

"Ever misread a patient's chart? Especially if you were tired and looking at numbers?"

"We all have."

"Absolutely, although there are some who will look you in the eye and swear it's never happened to them. But this is a human trait, not just a medical malady. Let me give you a frightening example from our airline friends. Back in the late '80s at DFW airport in Dallas, a Delta Boeing 727 was taxiing out for takeoff on an otherwise clear day. Now, at that time, Delta had bucked the rest of the airlines in refusing to institute training courses for their pilots that would erase the barriers in communication and get rid of the cultural atmosphere that killed Captain van Zanten and 582 others. Their chief pilot even appeared on a NOVA production on PBS about that time all but sneering at those crew resource management courses and saying in response that Delta was a 'captain-oriented airline' that justifiably expected their captains to decide what was best. Oh, yes, they had checklists and specific procedures, but their captains could alter them or deal with them most any way they saw fit, to some extent like most doctors are allowed to do. So this captain and two subordinate pilots are headed out on a routine flight with a moderately full load of passengers. The first officer has taken on the role of social director, chatting rather constantly with the captain, the second officer, and a flight attendant who came in for part of the taxi-out sequence, and while the captain joins in occasionally, he does nothing to quiet his copilot down and keep them focused on the job at hand. Some so-called non-pertinent chatter in the cockpit is normal, but on this day all the cockpit duties — including the reading of the checklists and setting of flight controls — is being done against the constant background of the copilot's talking. Now, when they get to the before takeoff checklist, in most cockpits the second officer reads 'Flaps,' and the pilot positioning the flap position lever for takeoff responds by saying '15, 15, green.' You know what flaps are, Will?"

"Things on the wings, I guess."

"They're big panels that slide out of the trailing edge of the wings and droop down to let an otherwise high-speed airplane take off and land at slower speeds. In flight they pull them back in and the wing gets, I don't know, more slippery and faster. Now a Boeing 727, which has three engines, can take off just fine with the flaps retracted, provided the pilots accelerate the airplane down the runway some 25 knots faster than normal.

But for the usual takeoff, the trailing edge flaps are in what they call the 15-degree position, both an outboard set on each wing and an inboard set. Also, there is a type of flap on the front of the wings called leading-edge devices, and when the trailing edge flaps are at 15 degrees, the leading edge slats have to be extended. When that's the case, they get a green light on the forward panel and two gauges — one for the outboard and one for the inboard trailing edge flaps — and they both have needles pointing to 15. So this crew is on the way to the end of the runway, the captain calls for the 'before takeoff' checklist, the second officer hits the item about flaps and calls out 'Flaps,' then looks forward and reads the gauges, seeing 15, 15, green. The first officer — also known as the copilot as I mentioned in the KLM story — looks over and reads out loud the same indications and says on the voice tape, '15, 15, green.' Now the captain can be heard shifting position in his seat to lean over and he, too, verifies that the flaps are set to 15, 15, green. Now, you know how difficult it is in an OR setting to get two physicians to verbally confirm anything, and here we have three thoroughly professional pilots who have visually confirmed — and one who has verbally confirmed — that the flaps are in the proper position for takeoff using a rotation speed of about 146 knots. They get their takeoff clearance, get on the runway, push up the power and start accelerating. At 146 knots the copilot calls 'Vee one and vee R,' which is their normal callout to rotate the nose up, and the captain pulls on the yoke, but the main gear is stuck to the runway. He pulls harder. They're still on the ground. Alarmed now, he pulls even more until the big jet's tail skid strikes the runway as the nose finally gets high enough for the aircraft to get airborne. But they can't climb, and suddenly the middle engine — which is fed by airflow coming over the top of the fuselage — doesn't have enough air, since the body angle of the jet is so severely nose up. The middle engine begins to stall — they call it a compressor stall — and lose power. Almost a third of their thrust is now essentially gone, and with all three pilots completely clueless about why it's not flying, the airplane comes back to the ground, rockets off the end of the runway at well over 130 miles per hour, bangs across a drainage canal shearing the landing gear off and breaking the airplane's fuselage in three places. It comes to a halt, fire breaks out, and 18 passengers lose their lives.

"All three of the pilots survive, and when the NTSB interviews them in the hospital, all three confirm everything was properly set for takeoff. But when NTSB investigators look in the still-intact cockpit, the reason they couldn't get off the ground rotating at 146 knots is painfully apparent: Despite all the captain's efforts to change the procedures to make things more safe, their flap handle is exactly where it was when they took the runway, in the fully retracted position. Remember that what we're talking about here is human perception. Three highly qualified, highly capable airmen very motivated to be safe, had looked at the same two gauges and that single light and saw what simply wasn't there. Three of them! Instead of 15, 15, green, the gauges read 0, 0, and there never was a green light. Further, the captain had failed to provide enough leadership to keep his crew focused and he did nothing to quiet down the copilot on the long taxi out from the gate to the runway. That's pretty much the equivalent of a surgeon who comes in to do his procedure without making any attempt to guide or even interact with the team as its leader. Now, just on the basis of the 15, 15, green mistake made by all three, you study this accident and you can't help wondering how any physician could be so arrogant as to think that he or she could be free of the same propensity for reading a gauge wrong, or seeing something expected that isn't really there. Bottom line, Will, is that as humans, we do not perceive things perfectly, and when fatigue, distraction, anger, or pre-disposition among other things, get in the way, we're capable of misperceiving just about anything. But the larger tragedy is that in medical practice we are taught to *assume* that no such propensity exists. We do not build our systems and procedures to expect such mistakes, yet such mistakes happen every day, as any honest anesthesiologist can confirm."

"All three made that mistake? That's amazing! Any idea why?"

"Yes. See, that's the beauty of using aviation accidents as examples, because they get investigated so well there's little if any doubt about precisely what happened or why. Totally unlike our medical accidents, the details of which are usually cloaked in secrecy and litigation for years, even within our own hospitals. What happened in Dallas is simple. The copilot was talking so much about unimportant things that when a radio call came through just as he was reaching for the flap lever he got out of sequence and failed to move the lever. In fact, the checklists were designed to catch that potential error. But the checklist backup didn't work, partly because the captain had failed to quiet down the talkative copilot and guide his crew on focusing on the job at hand, and partly because — using the latitude that Delta gave its captains at the time — the captain wanted all three pilots to listen and respond to the major checklist items such as 'flaps.' In fact, the crew had responded to the 'flaps' item so many more times than normal that it had become a mantra — almost a chant — rather than a checklist. They became so used to looking at the forward panel and seeing 15, 15 green, their expectation mentally blocked reality. The misreading of the flap position occurred because they were human, and humans are incapable of perceiving everything correctly."

"I can certainly add some stories on the dangers of assumption. For instance, that awful occurrence in Indianapolis in 2006 that killed three babies."[12]

"In Indianapolis?" Jack asked.

"Yes. In the headline version, three premature babies died when they were injected with doses of the adult version of heparin at roughly 1,000-times the safe dosage for an infant. What really happened, though, was a study in systemic error, and a classic example of assumption."

"I recall the case, now," Jack said. "A pharmacy technician inadvertently stocked the Pixus with adult vials of heparin instead of the pediatric Hep-Lock."

"That's right; Hep-Lock is a much lighter blue. Yet, up to five separate nurses, doing routine duties under the normal pressures of too much work and too little staff, pulled the vials from the drawer assuming they were the same ones that were always there, and the only ones that should have been in that drawer. They weren't. It wasn't misplaced trust that prompted the nurses, by the way, to not check any further than the correct drawer.

Trust is where you make a conscious decision that you can depend on something having been done. This was pure assumption."

"Absolutely. Yet it had happened before, as I recall."

"Good memory. Yes, they'd had two similar incidents with the very same Hep-Lock versus heparin mix-up in 2001, but none of the affected babies died. And, at Cedars-Sinai Medical Center in Los Angeles just recently the same exact thing happened yet again.[13] This time, because it imperiled the infant twins of actor Dennis Quaid, the media was all over it without understanding that the most important aspect of the story wasn't that a nurse made a mistake or even a hospital made a mistake, but that what is supposedly the world's best medical system cannot learn from its own mistakes across the nation. Why hadn't the systemic problem been fixed at Cedars after the Indianapolis tragedy? Because we're still more of a cottage industry than a unified international force of healthcare institutions determined to learn from one another's mistakes and never repeat them."

"That," Jack said, wagging his finger at the ceiling, "is the result of practicing medicine without a collective memory. We make the assumption that we've incorporated the lessons learned elsewhere, but that assumption is ludicrous because we have no system for doing so. In fact, flawed assumptions are at the heart of most such accidents. I've studied a lot of closed-claim insurance files from medical disasters, and I never saw a single one in which a flawed assumption of one sort or another wasn't a contributing factor. And take your experience last night. What did the ER doc do when he picked up only part of the chart?"

"He assumed it was all there, or at least assumed there wasn't anything else important to check."

"Right. And what did the nurse assume?"

"That the doctor had fully taken into account everything pertinent, including the warning sticker about allergies, which she assumed he'd seen."

"You're getting the picture. But here at St. Michael's, because we changed our culture to *expect* misperceptions and bad assumptions as the norm, the nurse had an additional chance to discover that previously flawed assumption. The prior assumption both she and the physician had made was dead wrong, and could have killed the patient. But with this new approach, she picked up the order, assumed that order was flawed until proven otherwise, and found that, indeed, this time it was. So the point is this: Making positive changes in a hospital system in order to prevent medical errors is what we need to do in every instance, but we have to be alert for overconfidence. Just making a change in a complex system is not enough. We have to live with, and work with, the changed system and make further adjustments, all of which requires teamwork and communication. Otherwise, unwarranted overconfidence can creep in now that all the problems are solved. One of the greatest generators of medical error is the fact that we expect everyone to do his or her job flawlessly, but even when we institute patient safety double-checks and other methods, we then make the huge mistake of assuming that everything has now been done right. How do you achieve true patient safety and get to where the aviation industry is with nearly zero accidents? By changing the culture into one that assumes everything will always be screwed up and dangerous until proven otherwise."

"And you mentioned communication?"

"Flawed communication is the bedrock-basic human malady that enables most medical mistakes. I've got a lot of examples for you, but I'm late delivering you to the ICU." Jack was already pushing back from his desk and heading for the door, but he stopped with his hand on the knob and turned back to the younger physician.

"One other thing. Are you free for dinner this evening?"

Will laughed in response. "I don't know. Am I?"

Jack laughed as well. "Well, I hadn't planned on locking you in the hospital tonight, so how about joining me for dinner around 7 p.m.? I'll find you when you're out of surgery and Alice is through talking."

"I'd appreciate that," Will replied, preceding Silverman out the door, "but I wouldn't want to take an evening away from your family."

Will could see a cloud cross the CEO's face. "My kids are on their own, Will, and I'm a widower. Basically these days I'm just married to St. Michael's. The company would be welcome."

"In that case, I'll look forward to it."

There had been a passing flash of sadness in his tone, but Silverman recovered just as rapidly and was now leading the way down the corridor with a brisk step.

Everyone has at least a few sad stories, Will thought, following the senior physician and wondering ever so briefly whether Silverman would understand if he ever heard the details of what had really propelled this quest.

No need to talk about it, Will told himself, feeling the old familiar flush of embarrassment.

Will's Notes:

1. Since human infallibility is impossible, the only chance to keep human errors from hurting patients is by creating collegial interactive teams (CITs).

2. CITs can't be effective without mutual caring and support.

3. CITs can't be effective unless all members of the team achieve barrierless communication.

4. There can be no barrierless communication if the team culture allows leaders to regard ideas, suggestions, proffered opinions and even diagnoses as unacceptable challenges to the leader's authority or ability.

5. There can be no barrierless communication if the culture successfully discourages subordinates from speaking up, regardless of the reason.

6. There can be no barrierless communication if the team leader's control is based on hierarchical snobbery, defensiveness, etc.

7. Regarding all medications as lethal unless proven otherwise has the potential to drastically reduce medication disasters based on assumption.

8. Having a team thoroughly invested in the outcome of their care is highly effective. The process is endlessly change-able, while the desired outcome the process is designed and

continually redesigned to achieve is singular and simple:
The best possible outcome for the patient.

9. Hospitals have traditionally been designed like "farmer's markets," with the landlord having little or no control over those who work under its roof.

10. The 3 basic ways humans fail, and thus the 3 basic tendencies a safety system has to address, are failures in perception, assumption and communication.

CHAPTER SIX

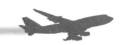

"Well, Dr. Jenkins, are you surviving your encounter with Knute?"

Kate Hefner, the charge-free ICU nurse Jack Silverman had just introduced, was glancing at the departing administrator and winking.

"I'm not following you," Will replied, confusion evident in his eyes. "And please, call me Will."

"I will, Will," she chuckled. "No, I was referring to our version of Knute Rockne. You remember, the legendary football coach at Notre Dame?"

"Oh, of course."

"I mean, we love Jack, but we have to hit him with a fire hose every now and then to keep his enthusiasm under control. So, ready to round with us?"

"Did I keep you waiting?"

"Yeah, and quite seriously we used the time to great advantage. But let's get moving. And I'm Kate, by the way."

She turned and ushered him deeper into the ICU where five men and four women were waiting.

"Let me introduce all of us first by position, then by name. You guys just nod, we'll shake hands in a minute. Now, the method is important, because it's very hard to recall such details in a quick introduction when you're concentrating on memorizing names. First, I'm the charge-free nurse, which means I'm the traffic controller and overall first sergeant and I have no patients specifically assigned. Second, this gentleman is our case manager. He is an RN with a master's in psychology, and he was hired specifically for his demonstrated skills in dealing sympathetically and humanely with the families and lovers and significant others of our patients, and being their advocate. I can't tell you how effective his job is, but even so, it took some convincing to get Jack to make the funds available. But what our case managers do, and have done, is vastly improve the plight of families of ICU patients. In addition… sorry to go on about this but it's important… having a case manager means that much of the inadvertent interference that families inevitably cause is eliminated. His counterpart — who was selected for the same qualities — works the evening shift, so we only have eight hours a night in which this position is not active and on watch, so to speak. But one of them has the beeper every night and has to be within 20 minutes of walking in the door. The lady to his right is our pharmacist. We have three pharmacists assigned specifically to the ICU, and they provide coverage around the clock. The gentleman next to her is our respiratory therapist, who is the single most important member in guarding our patients against pneumonia. The lady next to him is one of our two intensivists, who are MDs, of course. Our intensivists, like our hospitalists, are direct employees of the hospital, although here that distinction, as I'm sure Jack told you, means very little. The fellow to her right is one of our four dedicated and very effective spiritual care specialists. And then the two women and one man you see next to them are our nursing team on this shift. They are our vital eyes and ears at the bedside. And last but not least is our scribe, who carries two voice recorders as well as his pen and pad. Got all that, Will?"

"I think so."

"Okay, team, this is Dr. Will Jenkins. Will, this is our team and they've all got name tags so I'm going for first names and handshakes only." She ran evenly through every first name as they came forward to greet Will, and then formed a well-practiced semicircle around Kate Hefner.

"Okay, Will, you're next to Bill and for these rounds you're a full team member, and we specifically ask that you speak up immediately and participate in our discussions."

"I'll be happy to."

They all moved to the first bedside, Will noting how large the

ICU was compared to the ones he was used to. Kate greeted the patient, a Mr. Milos Karpagian, and his wife by first name. She reintroduced the team members to the Karpagians, adding the reason for Will's presence, and reminded them that the reason for the group visit was to bring the best intellect to bear on the plan of care. "And," she said to Will, "Milos and Maria Karpagian are full members of this team. We never, ever refer to a patient in the third person in their presence and there is never a dumb question."

Jenny, the nurse assigned to the Karpagians, briefed the basics of the case and how Mr. Karpagian had reacted overnight to a new round of antibiotics. She was interrupted several times, and Will noted how seamlessly the team discussed the questions and possible solutions before Jenny began the narrative again. On the second question, posed by the intensivist, Jenny herself spoke up, pointing out that Mr. Karpagian's platelet count was low. Not enough to be alarming, she said, but enough to make her wonder whether the antibiotics could be responsible. The pharmacist spoke up, providing the answer, leading Jenny to suggest that if the lower platelet count was expected with that medication and not likely to drop further, it might be prudent to stick with the same antibiotic rather than racing to try a new one. The intensivist told them about a new study she'd read a week before that validated Jenny's caution, especially with that particular drug, and the case manager asked the Karpagians what they thought after outlining the possible complications of experimenting further before knowing if the antibiotic he was taking would be effective. They indicated a willingness to wait another day, and the case manager explained to Will that they were understandably anxious to get Mr. Karpagian home because of a major family event being planned this month.

Laughing, he explained: "Our last daughter of five is getting married, and I want to give her away. Perhaps I *need* to give her away!"

The plan to stick with the same course of medication was endorsed and they moved on to the next bed, with Kate repeating her introductory procedure before another nurse began reviewing the case.

For a moment Will's mind flashed back to Aristotle's quote about the whole always being greater than the sum of its parts. What he'd created and led, Will thought, was a hospital of parts. Most of the same people, most of the same positions, but never had they operated like a seamless team. Here, each member was an equal partner in working toward the common goal of doing the best for the patient.

And that reality opened the door ever so slightly to a memory he'd banished for the day, and he mentally slammed it just as quickly. This was a time to learn, he told himself, not a time for recrimination.

Fourteen more patients and 14 more discussions followed. Each, Will noted, included enough information from the case manager about the patient on a personal level to remind them they were dealing with a living, breathing and often very frightened person.

Will fully expected everyone to disperse afterward, but instead, the team assembled in a small conference room while the scribe finished his notes and then took center stage, reading back each order and change for accuracy. Two small errors in dosage were caught, and at last the team members individually initialed the final version before heading out the door.

With the nurses back to their patients, Kate motioned Will to a chair behind what she'd called her command console.

"Thanks for the input on the article about infusion device failures, Will. That was exactly the kind of participation I wanted."

"I appreciate being brought in."

"Now, some other things I need to tell you about this: We didn't invent most of these procedures — they actually came from a rather brilliant bit of leadership in Seattle at Swedish Hospital."

"Really?"

"We'll steal good ideas from anyone if they help our patients. In this case, the nurse-manager of their ICU, June Altares, an RN, MN, had attended an IHI conference where her hospital leaders signed up for the *100,000 Lives Campaign*, and she decided to do far more than just endorse the principles. She went home and designed a way to make it work, and even calculated how many lives they were going to save by the very significant changes she made. First, she knew it couldn't be an effective interdisciplinary team unless there was an absolutely level playing field. Every member had to be able to speak up with no fear of being put down or met with disrespect or rolled eyes, and every opinion had to be given equal weight and consideration. They all became the patient's advocate. But more than that, they assigned dedicated pharmacists who were delighted to be able to share expertise many physicians seemed to want to discount. And, they covered the spiritual aspect as well, and provided each patient with an advocate and protector. By making those changes, she altered the paradigm and the results — the metrics. We adopted that model, and that success, here at St. Michael's and it fit like a glove within the larger interdisciplinary and cooperative team approach Jack was building."

"Very encouraging."

"Oh, there's more. We encourage, and even compensate, our people for using our experiences as the basis for medical papers. We're not quite a 'publish or perish' outfit like some universities, but we've generated so far over two dozen peer-reviewed papers on our methods hospitalwide, with many more to come."

"How on earth? We're talking about generically overworked people to begin with, right?"

"Yes, but what we've done here is hire a retired researcher who's an expert in producing and getting such papers published, and he does most of the work in setting up a team of grads and post grads from affiliated universities to work with and assist our staff physicians and nurses and pharmacists. Most professionals who would like to produce a study or a paper are intimidated by the process. We demystify the process and make it relatively painless, leaving them only the hard work of reasoning through and understanding the data. It provides esteem for the physicians and nurses, recognition for the institution and credits for the grad students. A win-win all around. It also helps immensely to have such published validation when you're trying to change a culture and you run into unenlightened CEOs and boards whose first question is always, 'How much will this cost?' versus, 'How effective will these changes be?'"

"I imagine there *is* considerable cost, though, correct?"

"Not in the final analysis, no. Save one life, eliminate one major lawsuit and recovery, one major boosting of insurance premiums and the attendant loss of community image and trust, and you've paid for 10-times what it costs. But you have to have leaders with a backbone who will hire two or more additional pharmacists, and hire intensivists as direct employees, not to mention our case managers. Then they have to peel enough funds away to knock out a few walls and create twice the normal ICU space. Did you know — you probably do — that there is a very fresh study which shows that of all the performance obstacles in ICUs that contribute to mistakes — missed communications, and the stress of staff and patients alike — a noisy work environment accounts for 46 percent, a crowded environment accounts for 36 percent, and insufficient work space for just paperwork accounts for 26 percent? The average ICU is terribly undersized, so we fixed that, and Jack didn't blink. The board did, but he stood firm and we ate up a few private rooms to get our ICU out of that syndrome of crowded, noisy inefficiency."[14]

"Impressive."

"There's more to tell you. What Swedish Hospital's model helped teach us was that the way to greatly reduce some of the ICU's principal enemies — especially ventilator-associated pneumonia — was by instituting what they called, and we now call, 'bundles.' These are procedural groupings — specific methods of doing things that are not allowed to vary, and in which no step may be skipped. Let me just hand you an explanation by Kathleen Bartholomew, another RN, MN, and a real force for change at Swedish as a nurse-manager before she started lecturing and writing books."

Kate handed over a single sheet of paper and indicated Will should take the time to read it before they continued:

Ventilator bundles and central line bundles alone are expected to save 34 lives at Swedish's intensive care units. A ventilator is a respiratory machine used in the ICUs to help a patient whose ability to breathe is compromised. A "bundle" is a collection of specific practices or process steps grounded in solid science with the goal of improving outcomes. For example, the "vent bundle" contains four elements: elevate the head of the bed, give medications to prevent blood clots and peptic ulcers, interrupt the patient's sedation, and assess the patient's readiness to wean off a ventilator daily. Compliance with these practices was measured, and unless all four elements were present every day, the audit score was zero. This "all or nothing" methodology improved patient outcomes tremendously. Pneumonia is a common complication of patients who are on ventilators. By implementing the vent bundle, the number of patients with ventilator associated pneumonia decreased by 68 percent — from 23 patients in 2004 to five patients in 2005. In addition, Swedish gained national recognition for the most significant improvement of any hospital by the Institute for Healthcare Improvement (IHI).

"Central Line Bundles" were also implemented in the intensive care unit, and of all the patients in the ICU, 48 percent have central venous lines. Bloodstream infections caused by central lines have a high mortality rate. The key to this bundle is appropriate insertion of the line. Following the Centers for Disease Control and Prevention recommendations, the nurses made a checklist so that all of the necessary supplies were on the cart along with an insertion checklist. A company was then engaged to make a central line kit, complete with an instruction sheet to standardize this process. Integral to the success of these measures was the feedback from nurses. June Altares said, "We kept changing the process based on the barriers that staff noted, so the process is staff-designed." These huge accomplishments in the ICU in 2005 are a tribute to evidence-based practice.[15]

"That *is* impressive, Kate. You've instituted checklists and bundles everywhere?"

"Don't get the wrong impression, Will. We are not engaged in reducing medical practice to checklists. As you well know, it's far too complex to pre-ordain every possibility and provide pat solutions. But the majority of health care has used that one fact — the complexity and subjectivity we deal with — as reasons for rejecting checklists and bundles and carefully assembled procedures. In reality, though, the approach that works can best be described, I think, like this. We work hard to do two things: Institutionalize and standardize those procedures that we know work best, and reduce variables in practice and response when those variables do nothing to contribute to the quality of decision-making of physicians and nurses. Are you familiar with the aerospace concept of standardization?"

"Absolutely. I know that checklists are only part of that process. Pilots, for instance, go through the precise same sequence in setting up their cockpit every time. They call it the cockpit flows, and they teach each crew position — captain, copilot, flight engineer — a flow sequence they use to set up the switches before a flight."

Kate was nodding. "That takes away the need to reinvent the wheel every time they go out to fly, just like going through a pre-op checklist removes our need to reinvent the OR setup and the pre-anesthesia contact with the patient with every case. Those elements that are routine are checklist and standardized-procedure territory, just like in here. When a bed is empty, we go through a checklist in making sure it's ready for the next patient. Simple, easy, and flawless if followed the same way every time, and procedures don't drain cognitive brainpower."

"I'm still very impressed by the story of how everyone came together and used those bundles, here and in Seattle."

"Yes, but I want to make sure you understand why they were able to craft them in the first place. See, that's the rest of the story. In addition, their success in Seattle involves their quest to standardize and distill methods down to a collection of highly vetted procedures that really work. And then they work hard to achieve 100 percent buy-in and minimize, if not eliminate, variations from those procedures. None of that would have been possible without solid and dedicated teamwork. See, at first, they were unable to write procedures that fit all circumstances. They had to work as a team to test, redesign, and retest their ideas until they had the right mix. And it's not just the teamwork — it was having a manager who recognized that the success of the effort would depend on it being user-designed. What they distilled into an action plan works so well, and can be changed so effectively, because it wasn't just handed down from on high. Rather it was the whole group working together —

physicians, nurses, everyone — in a daily process of refining how to create these bundles, that made them effective and universally accepted.

"Let me give you an example of why this was so important, this working the procedure back and forth until it's the right one for everyone to use. When there's a spinal cord leak involved in a post-surgical recovery, you can't elevate the patient's head, yet elevating the patient's head was one of the key elements in the first drafts of the ventilator bundle. It's one of those necessary steps that they believed could not be eliminated. In testing their work, one of the physicians just coming into the group saw this major conflict and got everyone back to the drawing board to re-craft the bundle until they had successfully taken that, and many other variables fully into account. Will, the point I don't want you to miss is just this: If everyone — RNs, docs, therapists, everyone — who was going to be involved in using those bundles had not been able to fully participate in their creation without rank or position getting in the way, this process would have failed and the patients would have suffered. See, as Jack says, it's not just the process of looking around and adopting the best of what forward thinkers like Don Berwick and his IHI have themselves assembled from many unconnected sources. It's not even the process that some brilliant and unsung people have achieved by turning some hospital department on its head and making seismic change for the better. What it takes to achieve the type of change we've created here is a hospitalwide agreement and the commitment of everyone to discard the old ways and construct an entirely new method of how health care is done. That new view has got to be 100 percent team-oriented."

"Why isn't everyone in the nation adopting this if it's that straightforward?" Will asked. "I don't mean to be contentious, but you make it sound so easy getting everyone in lockstep."

"It's not easy. Oh, the basic methods are straightforward and easy to learn. But what's devilishly difficult is convincing people to let go of the way they've always done it, step out from behind their professional and personal defensiveness, and actually focus on the common goal. I had a World War II veteran, a retired Army general who helped reconstruct Japan at the end of the war, listen to my explanation a few years back of how hard it was to change this hospital into a team. After I finished, he said our dealing with the deep suspicion of change around here sounded very much like his experience in watching the shell-shocked Japanese citizens slowly emerge from their shelters, and how long it took them to shed their distrust and join the American-led efforts to rebuild their country. The suspicions were so deep, the trauma so profound, the betrayal of their culture during the war so all-encompassing, that teaming with anyone to rebuild was anything but automatic. But they kept at it, because rebuilding the systems as well as the infrastructure without full Japanese participation would have been impossible. Essentially that's the same human challenge we faced here. Why isn't this universal across the nation? Because health care is full of shell-shocked professionals all hunkered down in their bunkers and clinging to the only things they've ever had proof would work. First, we have to get them out of their this-is-the-way-we've-always-done-it bunkers. Then we can work on instilling the common goal that so many have forgotten."

"That the patient's interests are primary."

"That doing the best thing for the patient is, and must be, the common goal endlessly recognized by everyone."

"You guys really do take this seriously."

"Will, I've been a nurse for 28 years. At first I loved it, and then I grew weary of not being able to care for my patients because of paperwork, overwork and busywork. I got weary of catering to the ego of physicians who couldn't even bother to learn my name and wouldn't take a suggestion from me if it was ordered by a federal court. And finally I became seriously depressed about the whole profession. Until I came here and had the amazing good fortune to help craft this renaissance at St. Michael's, I was ready to do almost anything but be a nurse. Now everything has changed. The excitement here isn't just in building something entirely new and watching it take shape and be effective, although I admit it's a heady experience. The excitement is in finding what we'd lost, what I'd lost — the ability to focus our hearts, souls and professional training on healing and helping people, and doing it together. We really do have a community of mutually respectful friends here, even those who've never met. It's fun, Will. Truly a joy to come to work here, and there are nights I'm reluctant to leave because I enjoy making a real difference. You understand what I mean?"

"More than I could ever tell you."

Will's Notes:

The high effectiveness of the ICU at St. Michael's is a result of amazingly good teamwork based on collegiality and constant communication. The team I rounded with included:

- A charge-free nurse;

- A case manager (RN w/master's in psych);

- Pharmacist (three assigned specifically to ICU);

- Respiratory therapist;

- Intensivists (two assigned);

- Spiritual care rep.;

- Nursing team of up to three (Each one's input and evaluation is welcomed, expected, and given);

- Patient and patient's family;

- Scribe, charged with accurate transcription and read-backs.

- Note: Basic model may have first been advocated by IHI. In any event, Swedish Hospital in Seattle was one of the pioneers in using it.

- Ventilator bundles and central line bundles!

NOTE: The best part of the story of how to construct such a system is the method of constant revision and rewriting until everyone's ready to sign off. They never stop fine-tuning, but they do it with complete consensus. "What it takes to achieve the type of change we've created here is a hospital-wide agreement to discard the old ways and construct an entirely new method of how health care is done."

CHAPTER SEVEN

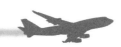

On the schedule Jack Silverman had put together for his visitor, lunch was listed as "on your own," and Will decided to take advantage of the time. He found an isolated corner of the cafeteria and was just starting to look over his notes when he realized someone was standing quietly by, looking for an opportunity to speak.

He looked up, somewhat startled to find a petite woman just under five feet tall who seemed all but dwarfed by the cafeteria tray she was holding.

"Dr. Jenkins?"

"Yes," Will said, getting to his feet, noticing blue eyes perfectly framed by honey-blond hair.

"I apologize for bothering you, and we could talk later, but Jack asked me to search you out." She extended her hand. "I'm Janice Morales, St. Michael's former risk manager."

"Former?"

"We abolished the title, and made up a new one. Now, I'm the chief safety officer."

"Please, sit down," he said, gesturing to a chair. "I'm just trying to absorb what makes this place so different, and it's a steeper learning curve than I thought."

"You have no idea," she laughed, stopping abruptly. "Well, perhaps you do."

"Tell me how your position differs from the traditional risk manager?"

"Gladly. In a nutshell, a traditional risk manager is the one who handles sentinel events, tries to identify and minimize risks in the organization, works with incident reports looking for bad trends in the data, such as infection rates, and generally tries to warn the captain where the icebergs are. Too often, of course, the risk manager's voice is too small to be heard on the bridge, to torture the metaphor."

"And, what does the St. Michael's chief safety officer do?"

"First, I'm a vice president and I report directly to the CEO, and I have authority to stop the production line, so to speak. Well, actually, everyone here does. But secondly, I don't just sit by myself and analyze data. I'm always organizing teams to face the fact that we constantly backslide into assuming we've got all the bases covered. You might say I'm the anti-assumption police. When we start thinking we're near perfect, I'm the spoilsport who comes riding in with the data — national or local — to prove that we're one assumption away from disaster. I understand Jack told you about our see-saw philosophy?"

"Ah, he didn't mention anything by that name."

"Okay... remember the see-saw you played on as a kid?"

"Sure."

"If you and the kid on the other end were roughly the same weight, it worked really well. That's because the thing was balanced about in the middle, right?"

"Yes."

"Okay, what if instead of putting the pivot hardware at the 50-50 point, where 50 percent of the board is on each side, you put it on the 90-10 point? In other words, 90 percent of the board is on one side of the pivot, and only 10 percent on the other side."

"You'd need a really fat kid to balance a really thin kid."

"True, and that's the lesson for all of us regarding assumption. We've created an amazing commonality of teamwork and mutual respect around here, facilitating a level of communication and collegiality I've never experienced in health care. We've accepted our own propensity for making mistakes and needing each other. But we have a human tendency to assume that now nothing can go wrong. So, for instance, we start a surgical procedure by making the assumption that there is a 90 percent probability nothing will go wrong, but we're still intelligent enough to know that there's maybe a 10 percent chance that something will. So we delude ourselves into thinking we're on guard. We tell ourselves we're watching for that 10 percent, but in reality, when someone sees a problem, they are now in the position of having to overcome the weight of the other side of the see-saw — that 90 percent assumption of normalcy. Jack tells me you discussed Tenerife."

"Certainly did."

"Well, what would that scenario have looked like if the assumption in that KLM cockpit had been 50-50? What if the captain, copilot, and engineer had been just as ready to acknowledge a potential major problem as the lack of a major problem? Of course, you'd also have to assume that their culture permitted subordinates to speak up without fear of offending the leader."

"I would imagine," Will began, watching her eyes, "that when the copilot received that strange clearance, instead of needing to believe an unprecedented one-word response from the tower was valid as a takeoff clearance, he would have told his captain to wait a minute, even though it meant correcting him a second time."

"And how about the flight engineer?"

"In a 50-50 environment, I don't think he would have convinced himself that his initial concerns were false, and that he should just, in effect, apologize and shut up."

"Right. But he had to overcome that 90 percent inertia that Jacob was right, he was wrong, and the runway was clear."

"Even the captain had to overcome his own inertia," Will added, "so in this kind of comparison, if the environment had been an equal expectation of failure, van Zanten would have let caution override his desperate need to leave and would have sought more information."

"Could be. At least they would have had a fighting chance. After all, he *was* the director of safety. The point is, we stop listening when we convince ourselves that all our safety concerns are taken care of. The see-saw philosophy overcomes that. We teach nurses in particular to be very aware of their, for want of a better phrase, sixth-sense. If something feels wrong, it more than likely is. I can't tell you how many times I've heard someone say, 'If only I'd listened to my feeling that something wasn't right, I would have stopped.'"

"So, you formally call this the see-saw effect, or philosophy?"

"We haven't come up with a hard-and-fast catch phrase, but that's the way I like to describe it — as a philosophy. And as the chief safety officer, it's one of my prime focal points, mainly because we've done such a good job aligning this entire team with the best safety practices and fostering barrierless communication."

"What kind of resources do they give you?"

"Well, for one, being at every board meeting and reporting directly to Jack, I never have to beg. By the way, I'm not at the board meetings just to answer questions. I have full right of participation short of voting. That was very courageous of Jack and the board, but it works. Of course, I'm careful not to blindside them with some new issue, but the board is very comfortable with my being a participant on any matter concerning safety and quality."

"How does your board define quality?"

"Excellent question, because we've grappled with that. Originally, one of the board members had decided we should adopt one of the prevailing models of assessing quality of care that produces metrics. What he wanted, not illegitimately, were datastreams he and we could analyze. He pushed us hard, and had us more or less wrapped around the axel trying to interpret the score that resulted from the measurement system we selected. Within six months we were spending more time trying to crib the results than use them for real improvement, and even our zealous board member came in one meeting and announced, very crestfallen, that he had suddenly realized the same thing: Most of his efforts in pushing us were now going to figuring out how to beat the system and get a better score — as if the score itself was the only thing that mattered. When Jack got through changing things, one of the items we effectively threw out was this measurement protocol. The main point is that in the process we broke cleanly, not only from the dominant point of view that quality of care can be scored and measured objectively, but from the way the tail was wagging the dog. In other words, we've learned to define quality as a living and breathing subjective analysis that changes day-by-day."

"But don't you need those metrics?"

"Yes, but meaningful metrics. It tickles me in a rueful way that anyone in medicine would talk about Six-Sigma standards when even the best of what we do barely approaches two-sigma. Such system improvement methods require a system to improve, and if you have no meaningful datastream on how you're doing, you have no hope of improving that non-system."

"You call it a non-system?"

"That phrase actually comes from one of the best books I've seen that deals with the business case for massive reform, called, as you might imagine, *Healthcare Reform Now!* It's written by George Halvorson, the Chairman and CEO of Kaiser Permanente, and one of the most compelling points he makes is that we don't have a system, we have a non-system, and it can't continue this way. He says that we must develop a real-time datastream if we're going to be able to improve our processes meaningfully, and he says that can come from nationwide computerization of patient records.[16] I think he's dead right. After all, quality is measured by how well we could have done clinically versus how well we did, not only in terms of outcomes, but in terms of process and communication and self-correction. We may save someone's life in a heart transplant against major odds, but if we got there through wildly sloppy and dangerous lack of coordination and poor communications, we did not do a quality job. By the same token, if we did a great job of process and outcome and the patient is still unhappy because our communications and interactions were not where they should have been, that means we did not achieve the quality we were targeting. It's everything, in other words, not just the things you can measure by numbers."

"You have a staff to do all these things?"

"I have six people working with me. I wish we could get CSOs with my level of clout in every hospital, but I doubt it will happen anytime soon, unless hospitals change their underlying culture. But let me tell you what else I have to work with here. First, I have a highly effective paperless, and blameless, reporting system that operates somewhat like the NASA Aviation Safety Reporting System in that it's completely secure. In fact, it's as secure as if it were fully anonymous. Only I and my staff can have physical access to the names of those reporting, and our jobs literally depend on never breaching that confidence."[17]

"Wait... why shouldn't it be fully anonymous? I thought that was the best method to get people to trust the system enough to use it?"

"It shouldn't be anonymous because an anonymous system lacks two very significant abilities. First, you can't call the reporting employee back to get more details, and that can be a fatal handicap in understanding the problem. And second, you can't fully engage the reporter on the beneficial effects of his or her report.[18] It's an arrow fired into the air with no knowledge of where it lands. People need to know that something is being done, because it encourages more reports and more fixes."

"I wasn't aware of those limitations. I've established an anonymous system before, and it wasn't very helpful."

"Well, it did take a while for our people to test our new system and realize that using it was not a threat to their career or even relations with peers and superiors. We make it very easy. You can go to any computer terminal and fill out a report, or even call it into a special number, and it takes less than four minutes, if that. Unlike the NASA system where, once the report is stripped of the reporter's identification no one can contact him, we always provide specific feedback so you know exactly what's being done. Many of our folks just waive the anonymous status, but it's there and it works."

"And it gives you an early warning system, right?"

"It's the backup warning system, and it's especially helpful for near-misses that someone is too embarrassed about to report in person. Fact is, we've become so good at talking to one another, even across departments and service lines, the vast majority of safety concerns are taken up directly, nose-to-nose, and solved right then. But for those who still feel nervous about wading right in, or who feel that it amounts to a confrontation — and they can't do confrontations — the reporting system picks up the slack and I can jump on it instantly. What we do here is what aviation has learned how to do. For instance, in the airline business, if a problem occurs on a Boeing 737 this afternoon that could involve safety on any other 737, by tomorrow morning every Boeing 737 operator on the planet will have been notified about it through a thing called service bulletins or airworthiness directives. They're told what to do if there's a fix available. There is no practical reason why we can't eventually do the same for the human mechanism. Here at St. Michael's, of course, we do. I even have an emergency network that I can use to send an urgent text message to every physician, manager, department manager and director about a suddenly discovered safety threat. I use it very judiciously, but I use it, and it's appreciated. We also issue a newsletter, but we're very careful not to include anything that isn't immediately usable information. In other words, some months it may be one page long, some it's five. We want the recipients to feel they need to read everything, not have to weed out filler."

"That's important. It's amazing how much we need to read. But this is all part of the goal of wiring everyone together in a sort of neural network, isn't it? I saw that phrase used in one of the papers Jack gave me."

"Absolutely. But while we've been working hard to solidify our own internal network, we also are very focused on helping the national problem by wiring ourselves into a national health care version of a neural network, especially with respect to safety discoveries and alerts that also heavily affect quality. Will, can you imagine how many lives could be saved and how many agonizing mistakes avoided if all of health care were as wired together as we are here? That's what great organizations such as the Institute for Safe Medication Practices tries to do with medication safety alerts. But we need much more, some method of wiring everyone together like the sort of emergency maintenance communications abilities the airlines have and depend on so successfully. Imagine, for instance, a situation in which a surgical team makes a bad mistake today in Boston using a fairly new procedure, a mistake that's easy to make but no one had warned them about. Then imagine that by tomorrow morning, everyone in health care who might need to know has been notified about it, knows how it happened systemically, and knows exactly what to do to prevent it ever happening again. That is my holy grail," she said, smiling.

"Jack used an interesting phrase. He said we're guilty of practicing medicine without a collective memory."

"So true. Aviation remembers every accident it ever had in excruciating detail. Now, having said that, aviation isn't perfect either. Sometimes just because everyone's notified of a problem doesn't mean everyone is going to fix it voluntarily. For instance, it sometimes takes an accident or well-publicized near-miss to get the Federal Aviation Administration off its duff and force it to change the rules. Many times the airlines will beat them to it. There was an infamous case back in 1989 where a huge cargo door blew off a Boeing 747 in flight, at night, south of Honolulu, sucking nine passengers to their deaths. The flight crew barely managed to get themselves and the rest of their passengers back safely. But it turned out that there had been a dress rehearsal for that accident involving a Pan American 747 two years before in 1987 when the forward cargo door of a 747 began gaping open in flight but somehow stayed on until the crew could return to the airport. Within days, both the FAA and the manufacturer realized a fix was needed for the 747 fleet, but due to the FAA's glacially slow delays in ordering repairs, the United 747 had not been touched by the time it taxied out in Honolulu."[19]

Will was nodding. "They call it tombstone technology in aviation, and we should probably adopt the same term. After all, we have to kill who knows how many before we begin to change our procedures."

"But, Will, whether we're talking about the Pan Am or United example, or, for instance, the Indianapolis preemies killed by mistaken administration of adult heparin, both types could be prevented by the type of system we've developed here. What if the Pan Am maintenance people had assumed that the same problem could bring down someone else's 747 and made sure the word got out through Boeing to every 747 operator, cautioning everyone to fix the problem immediately? What if those nurses in Indy had been taught to always assume that when they pulled out a drug for a preemie, it was the wrong drug, wrong dose, or otherwise potentially lethal until proven otherwise? If they had had a philosophy like ours and assumed the negative, not the positive, they would have carefully read the label, perhaps re-read it, looked at the color, and called for help if there was any doubt. Nothing would have been injected until they were absolutely certain. And even without that presumption, what if they had been trained to check the labels and the names as a checklist item that could not be bypassed or pencil-whipped."

"Pencil-whipped?"

That's an old aviation term used when someone enters false information about a flight or a maintenance repair in the log. You know, flight hours they never flew or inspections they never completed?"

"Understood. I used to get rumors all the time that many of my surgeons were pencil-whipping the time-out form."

"Again, in Indianapolis, every nurse would have caught the error in time, and the very first one to do so, if they were a truly collegial team, would have immediately alerted everyone else, including the pharmacy, and taken the responsibility for midwifing an immediate change."

"By the way, Janice, there's a small contradiction I need to clear up. When you're talking about the see-saw effect, you're recommending that everyone should have an equal expectation that there's as much chance of something significant going wrong as there is that everything will go right — in other words, a pure status of having no predisposition or prejudice in either direction. I understand that, but when both you and Jack talk about medication, suddenly the desired expectation is different. It becomes the absolute worst. In other words, you're supposed to expect that it *will* be the wrong dose, wrong medication, wrong path, not just be equally receptive to the possibility."

She was nodding and smiling. "I love a student who pays attention. Yes, that is a contradiction and it's purposeful. It's born of the reality that since the IOM report, we've made few inroads stopping major medication errors. Therefore, while most procedures and diagnoses can benefit from the 50-50 rule of expectations, medication is a separate problem and must be regarded for what it is: A potential killer each and every time. Take a highway patrolman approaching a driver's door in a routine traffic stop. That trooper's trained assumption is that the driver is ready to jump out with a gun and start shooting, and he protects himself accordingly with a long list of procedural steps and learned reactions. If the worst occurs, he's ready. Our trained assumption is that the wrong drug is moments away from killing our patient. If the worst occurs and it is the wrong drug, wrong dose, wrong path, our making that negative assumption and testing it means we'll catch the error in time. Like the trooper, we're ready."

"Janice, what was your toughest challenge when you put up the electronic reporting system?"

"That's depressingly easy. It was the low reporting rate of the physicians. This was several years back, and at that time — with all due respect to your MD status, Will — the physician group here was by-and-large the usual boys club, refusing to accept the idea that they could even make errors, let alone have a need to catch them. They followed Jack reluctantly in the reporting system because Jack is a force of nature, and these are basically very good people and good doctors. But so few of them used our system I had to make a major board issue of it, and Jack and I firestormed it through the physician group until they got the point."

"How?"

"By, excuse the analogy, rubbing their noses in the mistakes they were involved with that others had reported and they hadn't. We're not necessarily talking about errors they caused, but here would be a doc and a nurse side-by-side seeing the same problem, and who reports it? The nurse. Of course we never identified just who *had* reported it, but I basically told them their under-reporting was a professional embarrassment to their own medical groups, and that it had to stop. Slowly but steadily they all began to get on board."

"I'm sure it wasn't that easy."

"My story and I'm sticking to it," she laughed.

"I know you're right, Janice, and this is generic. We doctors tend to think differently."

"That's not an excuse, although I know you didn't mean it

that way. But, yes, nationwide it's a problem. Example? A year ago there was a study of 92,547 electronic safety reports from 26 acute-care facilities.[20] What percentage do you think were from physicians?"

Will smiled. "I'm feeling set up here."

"And you would be right, but take a wild guess anyway."

"Well, there are many, many more nurses than physicians in most institutions, so let me first say a ratio of one-to-six. Assuming, say, 20 percent of the reports were from people other than MDs and RNs, giving us a resultant figure of around 70,000, then — forgive my in-the-head math — but if it's 70,000 reports and a one-to-six doctor to nurse ratio, 10,000 of the reports should be from physicians, and that would be about 11 percent."

"Impressive calculating. So, you'd figure about 11 percent of those reports came from physicians, right?"

"Yes, if the numbers represented equal participation."

"Less than 2 percent came from physicians. That make my point?"

"Really? Only two?"

"Yep."

"Well, I do know you're right about us tending to develop a boys club. Even the female docs are members these days. I hate to admit it, but I certainly experienced it from the other side of the fence when I was running a hospital. The tendency among physicians has always been to protect our own — to share no evil, report no evil outside the professional ranks. It's like a twisted form of *Omertà*, the Sicilian code of silence, and frankly, it's protected many a bad doctor and some true butchers. I'm not proud to be associated with that history. Now, as to the reporting system — the one I helped establish at my hospital wasn't the same as what you've created here. It was wholly anonymous except for the professional category of the reporter. That's how we knew our physicians essentially refused to use it. The concept got twisted in their heads and they, in some weird manner, came to consider that doctors who used the reporting system were breaching some professional code, and instead were honor-bound to take care of their own problems. That might have been all right on innocuous things, but they seldom ever acknowledged their own mistakes and procedural shortcomings, let alone took care to change them. What I know personally, both as a former CEO and a doctor, is that our ridiculous tendency to be silent creates incredible levels of stress and mental distraction and upset among very good and moral people who know that problems exist but who aren't supposed to do anything about them outside of the club. It's hard enough being a physician these days without a constant moral dilemma. That whole cultural attitude — the way it was taught to me and the way almost all medical school professors still teach it today — is unhealthy and dysfunctional, and it's high time we bellied up to the bar and admitted it openly."

"Amen," she said. "And until you do, nothing in med school is going to change, and if med school doesn't change, we'll be fighting these same attitudes and dysfunctionalities 50 years from now, if not beyond."

"No, Janice, long before 50 years pass we'll be nationalized, gutted as a profession, stripped of all autonomy, and reduced to the level of a learned trade or a guild. We don't have much time left to get our house in order."

"Did you look at any of the license plates here when you came in, Will?"

"License plates?"

"Yes, in the physician parking places?"

"Ah, no."

"Well, take a look when you leave this evening. There's something unique on the license plates most folks in this country haven't seen in 30 years or more."

"What?"

"A caduceus. Physicians used to have them attached to their license plates or the frames that held them, not only as a matter of pride, but because police officers and citizens alike needed to protect their docs. It's a national tragedy that such expressions of professional importance to the community were allowed to evaporate. It's a national tragedy that fear of litigation drove our self-esteem underground. In fact, that fear began causing them to disappear decades ago, and by the '80s they were essentially gone. We've reissued them, and educated this town to respect what they represent. They still get speeding tickets, but they also get a lot more community recognition. It's a small thing, but very important."

Will's Notes:

- Met Janice Morales, former risk manager, now their Chief Safety Officer. She reports directly to the CEO. The position appears far more effective than any of the traditional "risk manager" roles, especially because this CSO has real power and access from top to bottom. The traditional risk manager has little or no power, and even the new "chief safety officer" positions popping up around the country usually are one or two steps removed from the CEO.

- The see-saw model is used by them to explain the off-balancing effect of a 90% assumption that all will go okay in a procedure. The point is that anyone seeing a problem has to overcome that 90% assumption, and if the person spotting the problem is not tenacious, assertive, and very sure of themselves, the information won't be passed.

- From the explanations I've been given, in-house reporting systems should not be fully anonymous because such systems do not provide feedback to the reporter. With no feedback and no reinforcement, other potential "reporters" are discouraged or at least not encouraged. In-house reporting systems can, however, be structured to fully protect the identity of the reporters.

- A very profound quote, supposedly from Jack: "We're guilty of practicing medicine without a collective memory!" Also recall George Santayana's admonition: "Those who cannot remember the past are condemned to repeat it."

- Interesting term: "Pencil-whipped." Comes from aviation but could equally mean falsifying entries in a chart.

- Even adjusting for the larger numbers of nurses, physicians use even the best internal reporting systems far, far less than the nurses.

- Look into getting a caduceus tab for my license plate holder!

CHAPTER EIGHT

It was the name that brought Will to a halt in the corridor. Even though it had nothing to do with Wayne Nolan back in Portland, whoever "Dr. Nolan" at St. Michael's might be, the sight of his plaque on his office door was enough to bring back the darkness of Will's worst day on the planet — a high-definition replay of the funeral and that final, awful glance at the man who had been his best friend.

In that heartbeat of a moment, Wayne Nolan's eyes had conveyed an anthology of pain and denial and breached trust that hit like a train. The body of Will's godson, Ronnie Nolan, lay in the casket before them, and that fleeting glance had conveyed a crystal-clear message from Ronnie's father to the man whose hospital had failed him: "I trusted you."

Will forced himself to resume walking, though the floor felt as if it were undulating in an earthquake. He felt sick to his stomach, and suddenly very tired, his memory replaying the bitter hopelessness that had accompanied Ronnie Nolan's autopsy and the reality that his father had been absolutely right. The failure was theirs. The loss of Wayne's only son had been completely unnecessary, completely avoidable.

The day's schedule was clutched in his right hand and Will glanced at it, forcing his mind back from the darkness. One fifteen p.m., it said, he was expected to join day three of a St. Michael's employee orientation course being held just around the corner ahead.

He ducked into a men's room instead and checked his appearance and his tie, trying to compose himself. Ignoring the circles under his eyes and the sunken, haunted look was going to be difficult. Whenever the memory returned with such force, it left him shaken and off-base for hours.

I'm doing this for Ronnie, and Wayne, he reminded himself, knowing his search for expiation, for forgiveness, was always behind this quest for the answers and the methods he was convinced he should have long since known. The "what ifs" ate at him at the most unguarded moments, and the worst of it wasn't just the fact that young Ronnie was gone and Wayne would never be his friend again. It was the sadness of suspecting that he could never adequately use the information he was gathering. Surely he wasn't thinking of another CEO position, he queried himself. But there was no answer to give, other than the weak justification that he would be a better doctor as a result of all that he was learning here.

But there had to be more he could do, even if his mind refused to go there for now. The quest for answers was all that he could see, and the learning curve was steep.

The idea of a five-day employee orientation course for new employees from janitors through members of the "C" suite was unheard of. Two days, maybe, or at the outside three, but never a full week. The expense alone boggled his mind, especially since there was no possible reimbursement for the lost time. But one of the many explanatory papers Jack had included in the package was the philosophy behind the orientation course: "On Friday at 5 p.m.," Jack had written, "we throw a party for our new members, but by that time there's been a big change. Monday morning they were employees of St. Michael's. By Friday at 5 p.m., they *are* St. Michael's, and every penny we spent is worth 10-times what we paid."

There was a copy of the schedule for the day on the rearmost table when Will walked in, and he picked it up and studied it for a second as he sat down, only to be asked to stand up again as the facilitator, director of staff education, Bette Reinertsen, welcomed him and introduced him to the class of 28 as if he were a visiting dignitary.

"Dr. Jenkins will be with us for this hour, and Will, if you don't mind, we're all on a first-name basis here."

"Absolutely I don't mind!" he replied with a smile, resuming his seat and thinking he could have phrased that better, and looked less surprised.

The subject was how humans fail, and as Bette Reinertsen began, backed by a carefully-done PowerPoint mix of slides and video clips, Will realized she was borrowing from a variety of industries, including aviation, the Navy and nuclear power generation.

"Yesterday we went very deeply into the three killers — the most consistent producers of human medical errors — perception, assumption and communication. I took you through the "15,15, green" accident in Dallas, encouraged you to use that phrase as a catch phrase at St. Michael's in a shorthand reference to anything we encounter or suspect as a perceptual problem, and we went into great detail Socratically about assumptions. We ranged from the lessons of Tenerife to four different medical disasters, each of which revolved around a lethal assumption. And Will, one of those, just so you'll be up with us, was the tragedy at Duke University Hospital a few years back involving a heart-lung transplant. Are you familiar with it?"

"Yes," Will said, shifting forward in his seat in response to the verbal spotlight. Indeed he remembered, since the tragedy and the aftermath had triggered so many bad, resonant memories in his own mind. "The lead physician on the transplant team, Dr. Jaggers, had a complex operation ahead of him and a team of qualified people, but somewhere in all the paperwork and the buildup and the procuring of the organs the assumption was made that the right blood-type match had been checked. Essentially, everyone assumed everyone else had checked the typing, and Dr. Jaggers assumed that, of course, the organs wouldn't have been offered if they weren't a match. Long story tragically short, they were not matched, and after a monumental struggle and a follow-up second transplant, the patient, a young girl from Mexico, died."

"Right. It was a classic example of how assumption can trip up anyone, and why our operating principles at St. Michael's are that if you make an assumption, even on the fly, make it in the negative or at the very least *test* it in the negative. Margaret? Give us an example."

"Okay, I'm coming off shift in the ICU and I've done my report and am in the elevator dying to get home on time and suddenly I can't recall for absolutely certain if I alerted my counterpart that Mrs. Black needs two units of blood in an order written on the day shift that wasn't ready yet. I worried with it for hours, so now I'm confused, but my habit pattern would have been to include it in my report, and I'm almost positive I did."

"In other words, you're going to assume you did."

"Normally, yes, before this training. Now I'd stop myself and say, if it can go wrong, it will, so the worst case is I forgot to mention it, and therefore if I make an assumption, it has to be in the negative. In other words, I'm going to assume I forgot to mention it because that is, admittedly, possible. Now, if it's something absolutely benign, like a magazine the patient..."

"Mrs. Black."

"Right. Mrs. Black, not 'the patient.' If it was something casual like that, not a big, big deal to Mrs. Black, and not about her medical care and I forgot to do it, worst case I can correct that tomorrow. But if it's important to her care, I've got to phone back or just go back upstairs and make sure. And I'll sleep a lot better as a result."

"Are you going to feel embarrassed?"

"I would have. I probably still will for awhile here, since it always felt like an admission of incompetence to highlight a mistake you made. But, I understand the protocol here would be for me to write it up the next day as a good lesson about how to respond when you're not sure."

"Why?"

"Well... of course to reinforce the policy, but more importantly — and I really liked this point you made — because it helps everyone else who reads such a safety report see that they're not the only human on the team who screws up occasionally."

"So it's a mea culpa?"

"No, I don't mean it that way. I mean if one other nurse reads my report and says to herself, 'well now I don't feel that bad about myself that I've made the same mistake in the past,' and further, 'and now I see I should have written my experience up and shared it as well,' then I've had a very positive influence on the system. I've reinforced the kind of constant experience-sharing you teach, for the best interests of the patient."

"Absolutely." Bette continued. "Now, let's talk about communication mistakes for a moment. Ever heard the phrase, '*I know you think you understand what you thought I said, but I'm not sure if you realize that what you heard wasn't what I meant?*' Do you realize that, and I'm being conservative with this statistic because some peg it higher, 12.5 percent of the time human beings speaking the same language and the same dialect with the same education involved in the same professional pursuit do not understand what one another say? In other words, we think we do, but 12.5 percent of the time, minimum, we get it wrong! This is why pilots have learned that since their careers, and maybe even their lives, depend on getting something right the first time in a radio transmission, they have to read it back to make sure it's accurate — and more often than they'd like to admit they find it wasn't. Sometimes that involves asking someone to please slow down, or to rephrase what they mean. There's this great story in the airline business of a senior Delta captain a few years ago trying to write down a complicated air traffic control clearance being read to him in high-speed New York staccato by an over-stressed controller in the JFK tower. Three times the controller rattles off the clearance: '*Delta Sixty-Nine cleared Atlanta as filed via the common one departure, except change route to read Richmond direct Anderson to the Fulton-four. Left turn after departure heading two-five-zero, climb to and maintain five thousand, expect three-five-zero within fifteen minutes, squawking two-five-nine-nine.*'

"Three times the captain asks for him to say it again a bit slower, to no avail. Finally, reaching the end of his patience, the Delta captain presses his transmit button. 'Kennedy Clearance Delivery...' he says in a slow, halting, southern drawl, '... do y'all hear... how... fast I'm talkin'?'

"'Roger Delta,' comes the snapped-off response.

"'Well... son...' says the old captain, '... that's about... how fast I can listen. Now... let's try it again a lot slower.'"

She waited for the laughter to die down before continuing. "How many of us in this room routinely read back telephone numbers or credit card numbers, or have had people do a read-back when you've given such numbers?"

Almost all the right hands in the room went up.

"Okay, and how many of you have had someone — maybe a doctor, a nurse, a pharmacist — issue an important order or request that if misunderstood could be a threat to a patient, and that person did not ask for a read-back?"

Again, most of the hands in the room went up.

"How many of our physicians in here never, ever fail to ask for a read-back?"

Two hands went up.

"Two of you, and there are six doctors in the room. Seven with you, Will. Okay, here's the deal. Read-backs insulate our patients against that 12.5 percent error rate. Any of you think a 12.5 percent error rate in critical communications would be acceptable to our patients or their families? If your son or daughter was lying in one of our beds in critical condition, would you want to gamble on that error rate? Obviously that's rhetorical, but I don't want you to forget for a moment why we make it mandatory at St. Michael's, for physicians, too. Especially for physicians, since you guys and gals are the captains of the ship. In a draconian environment I'd puff myself up and warn that it's a firing offense to not do that, but we don't do draconian here. What we do is say this is the rule we've adopted as a team focused on the common goal of the best care for our patients, and we will not — that now means you, too — will not give important verbal orders without read-backs, nor tolerate anyone purposely failing to uphold that standard. Someone makes a mistake and forgets? That's normal, and the backup system then becomes the person you're speaking to. Hopefully he or she will remind you that a read-back is needed, and then do the read-back. This is one of those no-exception forcing functions we've all agreed to make mandatory, because we know it prevents errors that can take lives, and just as with the other hard-and-fast methods I've gone over this week, I have a ton of data and peer-reviewed papers and anything else you need to convince yourself that this is beyond evidence-based justification. This just flat works, and it prevents horrible mistakes. This is also why we have the hard-and-fast rule that if a single nurse or pharmacist cannot read and interpret with certainty beyond a reasonable doubt what a physician has prescribed, the physician will be contacted immediately to clarify it. We will not rely on assumptions when assumptions could kill or imperil our patients. All these forcing functions and forcing procedures come from the medical leadership, which means physicians, nurses and pharmacists. Jack may be a doctor, but he didn't sit around and write them. We did so as a unified team, with one whale of a lot of gnashing of teeth and some posturing at times, but this is a sterling example of the best ideas vetted by experience. Remember, if it can be misread, misunderstood, misinterpreted, misquantified, or just plain missed, it will be. The way to guarantee that mistakes won't hurt our patients is to always assume the worst, expect mistakes, and use without variance the systems we've designed specifically to neutralize such errors. Remember also that there's a good reason in aviation for reading the phrase, 'Landing gear down and locked?' as a challenge on the before landing checklist in a cockpit. It's because pilots, like all we humans, will occasionally get out of sequence and forget to put the rollers out. Since landings are always a lot quieter and a lot less expensive if the landing gear is down, the slight humiliation of having to conform to a checklist is far less onerous than the humiliation of finding you can't taxi without maximum power and a lot of loud scraping noises. Not to mention the TV cameras you'll be facing soon."

"Bette, you were also going to go over normalization of deviance," a student noted.

"Yeah, remind me in a second. I'm on a roll here!"

They all laughed.

"Here's another part of the puzzle. When we operate as a unified team without hiding out in silos, it means two additional things. First, any and all of those procedures can be reopened and reconsidered and changed if we agree together they need to be, and we are always doing that! These are living, breathing systems and they need correction, addition, and adjustment, sometimes hourly. But what we *don't* do here is go maverick and change something without involving the group. Second, we're like a safety chain roping off a dangerous old well. When we all use the same procedures as if they were that safety chain

— procedures we've designed and agree are best practice — we succeed in keeping our patients from falling in. But if there's any break in that chain — someone not using an established procedure or method — then we compromise all the certainty we've achieved using procedures that we know work. And every department is a vital component in this quest. For instance, let's take housekeeping and dietary and human resources. Last fall one of our housekeepers was mopping the hall on Six West and heard a strange noise. Instead of doing the 'not my job' routine and pressing on, or just making the assumption that she wasn't qualified to judge what was happening because she wasn't medically trained, she opened the door, looked in the room and discovered a patient choking to death on a soda cracker she'd squirreled away. The patient had just undergone neck surgery and the cracker had lodged in her throat. Our housekeeper ran for the charge nurse who called a code and they managed to get the cracker out with a Heimlich maneuver, but only after the patient had passed out. No question the patient would have died alone and unheard had our housekeeper not acted immediately."

"Another example? Newest employee in dietary, working the evening shift, decides to double-check the orders because he's a bit disturbed by finding no system for cross-checking allergies with the class of dietary orders. One patient is listed as having an allergy to MSG, monosodium glutamate, and has had a no-MSG diet ordered, but he makes the worst-case assumption that this is a critical precaution and that our patient could be badly impacted if any MSG got through. He checks the list and all the foods seem like they conform, but just to be sure, he goes in the storeroom and starts pulling out ingredient lists, and guess what he finds? Four out of six foods that were on her diet are lousy with MSG. No one checked before, and the patient, it turns out, has been doing badly for two days as a result and no one knew why. He not only solved that problem, he wrote a solution, coordinated with the physicians and the charge nurse, and we ended up in a major realignment meeting to coordinate the menus and the food buying in the future. Larry? What am I describing here?"

"Well, you've kind of jumped subjects on us, Bette, but what you're talking about is responsibility and involvement, and that phrase from aviation — the one you were joking came from the fighter pilots — situational awareness."

"There's another word for it, too: engagement. Each one of our people I talked about was fully engaged and refused to consider the patients to be the responsibility of someone else. Each of our patients was and is their personal responsibility. That's because the attitude we try very hard to maintain — not just advocate — is that each of us, regardless of position and training, *is* St. Michael's. By the way, we don't just give an award, pat someone on the head and say, 'Good boy, here's a cookie!' when something like that choking patient incident occurs. That would be paternalistic and, in my view, demeaning. Instead we invite that member of the team to become a special ambassador of sorts to the rest of us and tell the story in great detail, including everything they were thinking, because the rest of us can learn important lessons from their experiences, their motivations and even their hesitations."

One of the group members had his hand in the air and Bette turned with a smile. "And that, *of course*, was the lead-in to what I need to tell you about normalization of deviance." She smiled at the casual ease with which they responded with chuckles and triggered a slide.

"Let me set up the normalization of deviance this way. We have a procedure in our ORs called 'time-out.' For those who don't routinely hang around in the OR, that's a very, very important protocol we use before a surgical procedure is started. The time-out checklist is run when the surgical team is in position and the patient is asleep. We didn't invent this, by the way. It's something that works very well when faithfully practiced, but in many hospitals where this was first tried, the doctors were offended and just rolled their eyes at it, called it cookbook medicine, and often just directed the nurses to check-off and sign the form if the surgeons didn't ignore it altogether. Many of the docs unfortunately took the procedure as an attack on their professionalism or autonomy, because, after all, a good doctor never makes mistakes, and therefore why would you need a mindless checklist to catch a mistake that can't occur in the first place? At St. Michael's, by the way, anyone, and I do mean anyone, can stop any procedure or function if they believe there's a safety problem or even an unaddressed concern. I'll admit that comes from the Toyota experience and from the U.S. Navy, but it's still a very important point, and hospitals such as Children's in Minneapolis and Virginia Mason up in Seattle have had amazing success empowering everyone with this approach.[21]

"You too, when we turn you loose next week, have the full authority of this institution, and all of us in it, to stop anything that's in progress, from a surgery to an MRI, or even momentarily suspend a code if there's a real safety concern. We use that authority very carefully, but each of us, regardless of position or training, possesses that authority and responsibility. Anyway, back to time-outs. If anyone tries to short-circuit a time-out here, the surgery will be canceled on the spot and there will be a lot of phone calls and a lot of group reaction. We've learned the lessons hundreds of airline passengers had to die for — that checklists, once written and deployed, are not optional. Believe it or not, before the late '70s, and for some airlines into the '80s, it was a captain's option how to handle checklists the company provided, or whether to even respond to them. Today you'd be suspended or fired in a heartbeat as a captain if you ordered your crew not to run a checklist precisely the way it was designed.

"That's the lesson for time-outs. When we go through that checklist, every item is called out and the appropriate team member checks that the item has been truly and faithfully done, and then reports it. We've gone significantly beyond the relatively minimal Joint Commission requirements. For instance, the anesthesiologists lean over and check their gauges and respond. The scrub nurse looks at and actually reads labels on critical vials and responds. If it's a heart procedure with an infusion machine, the perfusionist reads dials and gauges and visually checks the proper placement of his lines in and out, and then responds. No response is ever given from memory. If the checklist item asks whether a consent form is signed, the responding team member is obligated to physically look at the form and visually confirm that signature. By the way, the one big difference between our version of pre-op time-outs and everyone else's is that with each and every checklist item, the person doing the checking fully expects to find something wrong, and often does. Only after the attending surgeon and everyone on the team is satisfied that everything has been accomplished — including triple-checking of the patient's name, ID bracelet, whether the site is appropriately marked, is the right surgery on the right patient — can the procedure actually start. Now, what happens when we find something wrong? We do *not* treat it as an embarrassment. We approach it with the attitude that we've just uncovered another lesson we need to tease out in full detail and learn from. According to the Joint Commission, all hospitals should be employing time-outs, but it's not universally complied with.

"Most of the hospitals that employ time-outs, and that's fortunately a growing number across the country, are very reluctant to openly admit how many times their pre-op time-out procedure has caught mistakes that could have metastasized into disasters. Too often it results in an embarrassed scramble to correct the problem, red-faced apologies and no one reports anything. But our policy — much to the discomfort of our lawyer — is to openly share these experiences in great detail with each other. Yes, we take the names and the dates off the written versions, but even if we as a hospital run the risk of an occasional lawsuit, the value of what we learn from each mistake is well worth that minor risk. You see, each mistake caught by a time-out is not just a save for that day and that patient and that surgical team; it's an important message and relatively inexpensive one from the underlying system. Ignore that message and the problem it's warning us about will surface again, guaranteed, because it's a problem with the system, not just an individual Next time, if we don't adjust the system, we may lose a patient."

"Bette," one of the group interjected, "there's a concept in the law called the 'last, best chance' in avoiding an accident or injury. A time-out serves the same purpose, right?"

"Yes, it does. It's our last, best chance to prevent a tragic result in a surgical procedure by catching a mistake that has somehow slipped past all our other safeguards and procedures. Bar-coding at the bedside, for instance, which we do religiously, is also a great example of a last, best chance to catch a potentially harmful mistake that has wriggled past all our other barriers."

"And, Bette, this is to normalized deviance as what is to what?" Another of the class needled.

"I'm getting there," she said coyly. "Don't rush an artist. There was a valid reason for going off into an explanation of time-outs. Okay, so, were doing the time-out before a surgical procedure and the surgeon decides we can bypass and just check-off an item — say the one that calls for re-checking the ID bracelet of the patient. 'I read it when we wheeled him in,' the surgeon says. 'It's the right guy. Check it off and proceed.' So the nurse checks it off. Next day, same surgeon, same nurse, same type of procedure, and once again he vouches for the patient's ID check and once again she accepts it. That continues for the better part of a week until he also starts vouching for the check-off of the signed consent form, because he saw that, too. Nothing bad has happened with the first deviation, so she accepts this new one, too. Over the following months and the dozens of surgeries, three other items fall victim to the very same tendency, and each time — because nothing bad has happened from these small shortcuts — the nurse and the team accept the changes as normal. After all, they're saving time, right? This is now the new standard procedure for this surgeon and this nurse. They've normalized their deviations. Six months later, however, the surgeon one day speaks to his patient before the procedure and checks the man's ID bracelet without really paying much attention. Today the OR is really backed up and this is his fourth case, and if he doesn't get to the next one he'll have to cancel one of his patients. He races through his shortcuts, letting the nurse check them all off without really looking at anything, and as the doctor glances at the patient, he assures himself this is the same patient he spoke with before. Unfortunately, it isn't. The wrong patient has been rolled into the OR, and while checking the consent form and the ID bracelet alone would instantly catch the mistake and stop the line if the time-out check was faithfully followed, those last precautions have been removed over time and the surgeon's scalpel begins opening up the wrong patient for the wrong operation."

"I've read more than a few like that."

"Well, the lesson is that even small shortcuts begin the process of undoing all the safety systems we've put in place, and we can't afford to tolerate even one. Once we agree on a procedure, it must not be compromised in any way."

"You said that's how we lost the Challenger in the '80s."

"Yes. The classic case, and if you ever want to really immerse yourself in this syndrome, read an excellent book called *The Challenger Launch Decision* by Dr. Diane Vaughn.[22] This is cherry-picking only one of the contributing factors, but to my mind this is a crucial example. They weren't supposed to launch the Shuttle below a certain temperature, plus-or-minus 4 degrees, because of the brittle nature of the critical rubbery O-rings in low temperatures. But on one launch they went ahead and bent to production pressure to get the Shuttle in orbit and launched with the temperature at the low end of the tolerance scale. And, they got away with it. The next year it's 2 degrees colder, but rather than refer to the book minimums for launch, they applied the acceptable deviance scale against the previous launch temperature they'd used a year before and decided to launch again. Again they got away with it. Months later the very same thing happens, and they take two more degrees off the previous launch temperature and decide — over the objections of an engineer with the company who built the temperature-vulnerable solid rocket boosters — that they're still within tolerance. This time we lose the Shuttle and everyone aboard. And, there is a substantial school of thought that the loss of Shuttle Columbia in 2003 resulted essentially from a form of the very same malady — normalized deviance. As I say, there's much more to the story, but that part has always galvanized me."

Bette looked at her watch and walked to her laptop before turning back to everyone.

"Let me touch on what we just discussed and then we'll take a short break. First, we reviewed the three main producers of human error: perception, assumption and communication. We mentioned the Duke transplant sentinel event as a textbook example of a bad assumption triggering a disaster. Under the heading of communication errors, we talked about the 12.5 percent mistaken communication rule, and we discussed the mandatory nature of read-backs for critical orders at St.

Michael's. I mentioned our philosophy that if a communication can be misunderstood, misread, misinterpreted, or just missed, it will be, and that we must always assume the worst. Because of the need to expect poor communications, assumptions, and perceptions, we use various forms of checklists and procedures, and I went into some detail about the fact that all of those procedures are open to change, if necessary, by the group, but otherwise are not optional.

"Also, I totally reframed the concept of engagement and individual responsibility for the whole, which has a big role in minimizing communication and assumption errors, and I mentioned both the housekeeper who saved a patient from a killer cracker, and the dietician who solved an MSG allergic reaction, as examples. Also under the heading of engagement as a team and self-correction, we discussed the method of always reporting your mistakes and then becoming the teaching advocate for the lesson and any changes necessary, and we talked about the concept of situational awareness.

"Then, turning back to assumptions, we discussed our mandate to minimize assumptions, and to never risk a patient's welfare to an assumption. And we discussed the assumption-fighting time-out procedure that is mandatory here for surgeries, discussed the insidious process called normalization of deviance and the fact that at St. Michael's any member of the team has the authority to halt any procedure or action in the interest of our patients' safety. Bottom line, as Jack loves to say, is that only a team operating in total, egoless support of the common goal can catch and cancel the human errors that individuals and systems will always generate. One final note: When we say these things are not optional, we're dead serious. Breach these protocols once and we'll retrain you, and talk with you, and make sure you understand. Do it purposefully a second time and we collect your badge and show you the door, whether the union objects or not. We simply do not have the time or the capacity within the scope of our massive community responsibilities to put up with, or make exceptions for, folks who don't want to follow the hard-won template we've created here, and we simply won't try. So, as harsh as it sounded yesterday and will sound tomorrow, if you think even way down that you're not able to wholly and enthusiastically embrace these philosophies, please resign before the week is out. Okay, 15 minutes and back here, please."

With fresh coffee and soft drinks in the corridor, the group filtered out, most of them in animated conversation as Will approached Bette.

"Impressive method," he said, smiling.

"Let's say a proven method, Will. We revise it every time, but we've found it's far better to be brutally frank about compliance demands, because one bad apple in the ranks for just a month can really cost us time and focus and even morale."

"Do you test them this week, too, or evaluate them?"

"I didn't use them this hour, but did you see those little audience response handheld units on the tables? We use those without attribution through the week to gauge attitudes, and if I see more than one or two consistently negative attitudes coming through and I can't pinpoint who it is through classroom discussion, then I administer a test on Friday morning. Almost every month there's someone we ask to leave quietly before the end of the day, doctors included."

"Aren't you taking this a bit far? This reminds me of qualifying to join a church, or a specific religion."

"That comparison used to irritate and even upset me, but it doesn't any more because in effect, you're right. We're asking them to join a philosophy and practice it wholeheartedly. We can't maintain our progress if we start diluting the membership with non-believers. And as I said, we just don't have the time to mess around."

They headed for the corridor in further discussion, passing a gaggle of class members and two women in conversation, one who was saying that it looked like this was the place she had been searching for her entire career. She exclaimed, "I mean, the thought of being able to say, hey, this is what my patient needs, and have a supportive response from even the physicians is wonderful!"

Her companion, with her back to Will and Bette, snorted loud enough to be heard above the background chatter. "Yeah, like *that's* going to happen."

Will glanced at Bette who had her finger to her lips until they walked past.

"After the break," she said.

Will's Notes:

- The role of a 5-day employee orientation course in establishing a tight, coherent teamwork mentality for even the newest employee of whatever rank seems pivotal. It's a form of boot camp without the harassment, but using the same basic philosophy military leaders have used for centuries: Bind everyone into a common purpose and instill enthusiasm for what they can accomplish together.

- According to St. Michael's team, at least 12.5% of the time humans do not understand what they're saying to one another. I'm told, in fact, that many researchers have come to an even higher percentage. But add disruptions, fatigue, linguistic and cultural differences, and whatever the percentage is, it climbs alarmingly.

- Read-backs of critical orders or other critical informational communications (critical meaning something that if misunderstood could endanger a patient or practitioner) are essential to any patient safety program. Plaintiff lawyers in medical malpractice cases already know this and are ready to pounce on doctors, nurses, pharmacists, etc. who failed to use read-back protocols in incidents that led to patient imperilment.

- The basic rule in human communications expectation: If it can be misread, misunderstood, misinterpreted, misquantified, or just plain missed, it will be. This is a slightly more eloquent expression of Murphy's Law.

- The basic "time-out" procedure is another essential element of patient safety and must be imposed as a non-negotiable, no-variance procedure prior to all surgeries. More important, if something goes wrong and you've failed to do a time-out with everyone fully participating, including the attending, the medical malpractice lawyers will have a field day using that one fact to extract a huge recovery from an angry jury. Even in states with caps, a determined and angry plaintiff who doesn't care about the monetary recovery can seriously damage a hospital. Again, the lawyers know this stuff, so we'd better be doing it.

- Normalization of deviance is a profoundly important concept! I can see where my entire hospital was unknowingly adrift in terms of normalized deviance from standards of practice and best practices. We didn't institutionally have a clue there was even such a concept, let alone how to apply that knowledge to prevent the kind of disasters I was trying so hard to stop.

CHAPTER NINE

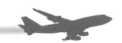

The schedule called for Will to head for the surgical suites at 2:45 p.m., and it was coming up on 2:15 p.m. as the orientation class reconvened. Bette had asked him to stay around for a few more minutes, and he took his seat again as she opened the hour by looking directly at the woman who had made the disparaging statement during the break.

"Okay, let's get real here. Who doesn't think all these great ideas and concepts will work as advertised?"

There was silence, and an increasing number of glances around as the participants tried to discern what had prompted the question.

"Come on, folks. Most of you are veterans of the health care wars. We have a new vice president in here, we have experienced nurses and doctors... and I've just given you a Pollyannaish view of a wonderful world that you've never experienced, right? So who thinks this is unbridled idealism?"

A little muttering, but no takers, and she bore in. "Even if it is idealistic, one of the basic premises is that we speak our minds for the betterment of the patient's plight, even if it is just to say that these great ideas are flawed or just naive, so it worries me that no one's speaking up. Didn't you believe me when I said there is absolutely no penalty for anything you discuss or opine?"

A tentative hand went up from a woman Will had already identified as a new pediatrician.

"Bette," she began, very much in control but cautious. "I... think all of us are a bit dazzled and we all hope all this will work, but we've never, as you said, seen it work, and we're new here. So... I guess our reservations are more of a 'wait and see,' than an attitude of 'it won't work.'"

"Okay. Wally," she said turning to the other side of the room, "you're our new member of the 'C' suite. Is this smoke and mirrors?"

A heavyset middle age man with a large smile shook his head. "I'm prejudiced, Bette, because the uniqueness of St. Michael's is why I'm here. So, no, I believe it does and will work, but if, and only if, everyone stays on the same page."

Bette turned back to the woman with the disparaging comment in the corridor, identifying her this time.

"June? How about you?"

"You don't want to hear from me," she said.

"Yes I do. Give us a reality check."

June bounced manically between uncomfortable and relieved, and Will could see the skepticism that had been roiling just beneath the surface finally hit a boil. "Okay, hey, look, no offense, but I wish all this would work. I wish it would, but I don't see how. People are people and about the time I get all excited and speak up on the floor — regardless of how touchy-feely everyone is in here — someone's going to 'slap' me back into place. That's nursing. We're professional victims. We're the bucket of crabs."[23]

"Sorry?"

"Well, there's an old story about a kid with a big bucket of live crabs for sale on a dock in New England, and a tourist tells him, 'Hey, son, you'd better get a lid for your stock or they'll be over the top and gone.' The kid says, 'Mister, you don't know nothin' 'bout crabs. They can't get out of there. As soon as one of them tries to escape, the others will reach up and yank him back down.' Well, that's nursing. The penalties for trying to think outside the box and help solve problems and stepping out of the mold to consider new ways of doing things always results in a stinging backlash. The others yank you back down."

"Wow. So you don't think it can change?"

"Well, let me give you an example from my previous hospital where they were all about openness and suggestions and working together. All wonderful until you made a suggestion, of course. One day, one of the sweetest, most dedicated nurses I've ever known watches a doctor using half a bottle of hydrogen peroxide on a patient's open wound he's redressing. After they're both out of the room she approaches him very respectfully and says, 'Doctor, could I speak with you about something new I learned?' He says 'Sure,' and seems to be friendly enough. So she tells him about an article she's read in a major medical journal that reported solid new research indicating that direct application of hydrogen peroxide in that sort of a situation actually retards healing and kills too many of the reforming cells. He listens, leaning up against a file cabinet, and then says 'Well, Barbara, why don't you get me the research on that.' She goes home that night on a cloud. Little ol' her has actually had something professionally beneficial to provide to an experienced doctor, and she really likes and respects this man. She feels like a colleague! She's up until 1 a.m. on PubMed pulling off the basic research paper and supporting articles and other research that might be useful, and she puts it into a notebook and prepares a professional analysis and summary, and tabs the pages. The next day when he comes in she proudly hands the physician the report, he glances at it, reads the cover, then puts it down on the nurses station and says 'Thank you, Barbara. Now, would you come in here a minute and help me with this patient?' She follows him into the room of the same patient he'd been seeing the day before, and he takes an unopened bottle of hydrogen peroxide, removes the lid and the patient's bandages, then keeps his eyes on her as coldly as possible as he pours the entire contents slowly into the wound, tossing her the empty bottle without a word when he's done. Can you imagine how she felt? She slunk out of there in tears, just shattered, and avoided him for the next three years. She'd flee and duck into a room when she saw him coming. The feelings would come back like post-traumatic stress disorder every time she saw his face. She never had another conversation with the man, even though she took care of his patients constantly. So, no, you tell me we're part of the team and can speak up and all that, and I'll believe it when I see it. I don't think the doctors can change, and I'm sorry for you doctors in the room, but that's how I feel. Experience is the best teacher." (Sadly, this is a true story.)

She sat down, shaking slightly and obviously upset as a hand went up.

"Yes, Rich."

"Well, I hate to hear stories like that, but I think the kind of abusive attitude she was describing can be stopped, and that the physicians themselves can put a halt to it, since, in my experience, the number of doctors that just have to be hateful like that is very limited.   But consider what drives a physician to be so nasty and small. This isn't meant to be a justification, okay, but a lot of docs are hurting and angry and defensive, and sometimes they just react badly."

"Sounds to me," Bette replied, walking closer, "like a physician harming a patient with a bottle of hydrogen peroxide is doing a lot more than just reacting badly."

One of the doctors raised his hand and she pointed to him.

"Bette, there's no excuse for that behavior — period. But there's also no excuse for having a staff of nurses so timid and cowed that they won't march straight to their nurse-manager and report the guy."

"So, the offended nurse should have had a tougher hide, right?"

"Yes," he said, realizing as she smiled that he'd walked into a bit of a trap.

"I won't exploit the obvious problem with your response," Bette continued, smiling as laughter rippled through the group. "The fact is, people are people, as June pointed out, and some people are going to be intimidated if we don't give them a system that energetically supports and protects them, and an ethic that makes not reporting such conduct unthinkable."

Another hand went up.

"There's an elephant in the room, Bette, and it's named 'money,'" one of the men said. "In nursing, for instance, staffing is a monster problem. There's a nationwide nurse shortage, and then you have hospitals that cut back so far on staffing that the remaining nurses are exhausted and practically in tears, unable to even take time for lunch. What's the idiotic reimbursement rate now from the government for hospitals, 28 cents on the dollar? That's societally insane, and I know St. Michael's has to absorb huge amounts every year from patients without insurance who, it turns out, are not mostly illegal aliens or the indigent. The people sucking up our resources with no money to pay are largely just working Americans who don't have insurance. Doctors, for their part, are totally confused and distracted about where their money is going to come from, and they're never sure whether capitation or some modified fee-for-service version is best. Some specialists reportedly have signed up with up to 50 PPOs at once! The craziness of this system cannot continue, but in the meantime the dollar drives everything. I mean, I'm impressed with Jack and the entire leadership here and I'm excited to be a part of it, but I'm worried — not that we can't come together with respect and work for a common goal, but that this hospital is a medical version of Camelot, and it won't last."

"You mean financially?" she prompted.

"Yes, I mean financially. So we add the extra people, and we pay for a week of this great training, and we buy the lifts for heavy patients, but at the end of the year, the books have to balance or the doors close. Does everyone here realize that in the year 1980 almost 80 percent of medical procedures were done in hospitals, and by 2000 that was down to 20 percent? 'If you build it' no longer means, 'they will come.' Hospitals are wallowing rudderless through a national hurricane of clueless decisions and governmental apathy, and most Americans don't even realize how bad it is. On top of it all, we're the only major industrialized nation that thinks health care is a business, an industry, rather than at the very least a form of vital public utility. Remember the incredible consolidation of the '80s, with for-profit corporations snapping up hundreds of hospitals in the expectation that everyone was going to make a killing? Thank God that kind of venture capital pressure has pretty much died away. But no matter how determined we are here at St. Michael's to stay our own course and provide a shining renaissance in safety and quality and staff happiness, where is the money going to come from?"

A male voice answered from a side entrance as Jack Silverman walked in with a smile.

"Not a thing this man said," he began, pointing to Rich and watching a sudden apprehension cross his face, "is anything but dead right, and well-stated to boot. Let me put all this in perspective for you, okay? Yes, the financial side is rough. We're a non-profit and we have to scramble as if we were a for-profit just to stay afloat. The distinction is almost academic. The country *has* lost its collective mind, permitting the sort of lopsided funding that hospitals have to depend on. The insurance situation by itself is a disaster in every respect, and we have a Congress only interested in playing politics with some of our deepest problems and playing stupid games with a tort system that can never provide justice in cases of medical mistake. Congress is wholly disinterested in the fact that this is a national crisis needing a moon-shot mentality to fix. Leadership is in short supply. But, so far, at St. Michael's we've kept the doors open, and with luck and great thinking by all of us, we will continue to do so. Not by my standing here saying that, by the way, but because we're reaching into our own brain trust as well as reaching to the community we serve and demanding teamwork from everyone."

Jack paused to pour some water and gulp it down. "One of the most dangerous truths in American healthcare is that we do not get paid for keeping people well and curing them fast. Many times hospitals and other healthcare systems have nobly undertaken to improve the health of their community in some way and succeeded, only to find that their revenues dropped measurably because of the resulting reduced need for treating the disease they were trying to address. George Halvorson has hammered this point home in the book you'll find on your reading list, *Health Care Reform Now!* The man tells it like it is, and while the entire country has got to find a wholly unique way of rewiring this backward system, we decided to do what we could here to lead the way. Let me give you an example. We've kicked off a major push to improve the health of the entire community in a way that might financially devastate us if we hadn't devised a way to rewire the whole relationship. In the next decade, the less the local population needs our services for serious things, the better off they and we will be financially. It's an amazing idea, but it can and will work. And it has, as its basic engine, an agreement with the community to change the law to provide us tax-based compensation for the number of admissions we lose over time to increasing community health, predicated on increasing drastically the effectiveness of our clinic-based prevention programs. In addition, we now ask for a 12 dollar per patient contribution for the indigent patient fund, and we ask the same from the community. This past year we paid for nearly 20 percent of our otherwise unreimbursed costs for the uninsured. Next year that figure will double because a corporate campaign is starting to help us and participate in the community's overall health. Businesses are going to match our patients' contributions. One of our X-ray techs thought that up!

"Now, one wonderful financial reality is that everything we're doing for patient safety and service quality is already showing up on the bottom line because of the following equation: Increased patient satisfaction plus substantially reduced injuries from mistakes that impact our patients equals less average length of stay plus greater staff satisfaction, which also equates to less staff turnover and expense, and lower insurance rates through our new and very effective self-insured status. In turn, all of that keeps our operating costs less than our income.

"Internally, when we find ourselves running out of budgeted funds in a particular area, we don't mug one service line to fund another, we get everyone together — including you front-line troops — and we go through beer, pizza, wine and ideas until we begin to find a way. Sometimes the collective decisions we come to are hard to swallow, but we've done it together, and in all decisions, we make absolutely certain there is no impact on safety, quality and enjoyment of practice. Last year we even eliminated a service line rather than let it be impacted by cutbacks, and we redeployed all the folks beneficially. And I'll tell you this, although we may have to make more tough decisions in the future, the one area we will never compromise is safety. Our chief safety officer's office and authority will be the very last door closed and the very last light to be extinguished if this hospital ever closes, and that's a pledge even the board has made. Another lesson the airlines learned the hard way: Compromise safety, and everything else crashes in the long run. Here's the bottom line, and I know Bette makes fun of my overusing that phrase."

Everyone laughed and Jack chuckled as Bette rolled her eyes at the ceiling and feigned innocence.

"The bottom line is that we're actively rebuilding the ship while it's sailing through very troubled waters. This is an institution in transition in a so-called industry that's both in crisis and transition. And while the long-range outcomes for both us and the nation are anything but clear, this we know for a fact: If we stick together and practice the philosophies that we teach in here and practice out there daily, if we'll depend on each other for answers to terribly difficult questions even when it seems at first there is no answer, we will not only make it financially, but we'll do so without ever compromising what we've built here and what we're practicing here. Our number one quality is flexibility to keep changing and adapting as we morph into something new. While we're doing that, we're also building and maintaining a neural network of communication between and among each and every one of us. At all times that will enable us to keep a solid grasp on those qualities we hold indispensable — qualities we know as a matter of certainty will keep our patients safe.

"What can you do? Don't join us thinking you're helpless. You have important new information we probably haven't considered. You may not have any idea how important your contribution is going to be, and hey, I'm not just talking to Wally, our new VP of Services over here, I'm talking to June, and Bill, and Jose, and everyone in the room. If you're pushing a broom at 2 a.m., you may have the one insight that saves a dozen lives. If you're laboring in assumed obscurity in the lab, you may realize something that all of us have been missing for a generation. Let those ideas slide by unconsidered and we all lose. We need you. And be prepared, because we're going to land on you like a leech, hungry for the serum of everything you know.

"But, let's get back to money for a second. I can't even begin to hold onto the financial helm if each and every one of you isn't at my side and in my ear and thinking for all of us. Think about the massive contribution of our X-ray tech, Jan Hoffman, who came up with that great idea for indigent funding. The next saving idea may come from you, but not if you let past experiences convince you that people and institutions and professions can't be changed.

"There is the way things were — such as with that hydrogen peroxide story I heard before I stepped in — and there are the way things can be. We have to support each other and make tough choices together, and most importantly — and this is one of my charges — we have to keep the power distribution even across the spectrum of St. Michael's. You are the keeper of my time, not my secretary, Cynthia. If you need to see me or talk to me, that's what's going to happen, and she knows it. She'll ask you if she should interrupt a board meeting or a something else, and *you* make that decision. Please be judicious, but I'm serious. We all work for each other. And, if we in the so-called 'C' suite make a decision directly or indirectly affecting your ability to provide our patients with the safest and best, we come to you for advice and ideas and help. We come to you and demand your best efforts in solving whatever we face. And we listen carefully to you. This is how we create not only the incredible safety record that has attracted accomplished men like Dr. Will Jenkins back there to come halfway across the country to study us, this is how the strongest possible network known to systems thinking is constructed. And this is how we can also help our nation, by continuing to be a flagship proving that things no one imagined possible can be done.

"I know I'm a cheerleader, but I'm telling you the unvarnished truth. Can I guarantee we're going to succeed? In being safe and smart and high-quality and a great and even fun place to work, absolutely! Although I warn you the price of joining us is our demand that you fall into lockstep and adopt our philosophy and enthusiasm. Can I guarantee in the long run that St. Michael's will be here five or ten years from now? No, I can't. I think we will, but neither life nor unions nor a great dedicated management team can make such a promise. So you're all taking a gigantic risk coming aboard. Actually, you're taking a monstrous risk for another reason: We're going to warp your mind. After you've worked here for six months, you'll never be satisfied with anything less."

He turned to the instructor and smiled. "Okay, Bette, enough of me, back to you. Thanks, everyone, I'll be in to spend the morning with you tomorrow. Write down questions tonight and be as brutal and direct as you want. We don't have time to dance around tough issues."

Jack left the room as abruptly as he'd entered and Will glanced at his watch again as Bette triggered another slide.

"Okay, we've got a video cued up to show you called *First Do No Harm*,[24] the first and second installments, which chronicle in a gripping fashion how easily a series of small errors can lead to a disaster when just a few people fail to stay engaged with the common goal. We'll discuss it afterward.

"But before we roll that tape, let me tell you a quick story to illustrate how devastating normalization of deviance can be, because we want you to be ever vigilant for the beginnings of any such sequence. Despite the fact that non-professional reading materials were never acceptable in ORs during a procedure, 30 years ago copies of the *Wall Street Journal* started making their way into the hands of bored anesthesiologists during long cases. Then magazines appeared, and 15 years ago, cell phones also appeared in some ORs, but just to handle emergencies. Around 10 years back, the use of cell phones by anesthesiologists during procedures was becoming somewhat depressingly common-place, and shortly thereafter, even laptops began to appear. Now, these are doctors, right? They're not going to do anything to compromise the patient. But in the space of less than 30 years we'd gone from no distractions to some anesthesiologists bringing laptops and cell phones into the OR, and stories began to circulate of a few rogue doctors day trading and running a web real estate business while their patients were under. That's why we're determined to never start down that road, even with the smallest of deviations."

Will's Notes:

Get the video "First Do No Harm," both installments. It's a powerful look at the clinical realities of all these aspects of patient safety and human communication. It was painful to watch, especially for me, but it's very good.

CHAPTER TEN

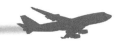

"Head spinning yet?" Jack Silverman's deep voice caught his ear from behind as Will Jenkins turned.

"Jack! I'm wearing out my pen taking notes."

"What do you think of the orientation class?"

"Well, first, Bette is impressive, but so is the material. As were you. Have you run metrics on the effectiveness?"

"With every class. We squeeze them hard, even six months later, as to what was good, what was useless, etcetera. The course content changes constantly. But to answer you head on, it's doing exactly what we wanted. It gives everyone the details of what our teamwork and open communication philosophy is, grounds them in the eternal fallibility of humans, and instills the reality in no uncertain terms that we mean, and will enforce, what we say about conformance to the procedures and guidelines we've spent so much energy crafting together. And maybe even more importantly, they come out of that course energized and feeling like they're not just a part of this great place, they *are* St. Michael's. Like Southwest Airlines people."

"Things can't be that perfect, Jack, in terms of the way new folks fit in."

"Of course not! Good Lord, Will, we're dealing with carbon-based units."

"*Star Trek* again, right?"

He chuckled. "You bet! Let me finish my thought, though, and then it's time to tell you why I keep mentioning *Star Trek*."

"Hey, have at it."

"We make mistakes, of course, and sometimes we don't find out for months that someone's a square peg in a round hole, and we still have to have a disciplinary function, but we do it differently. When we have a major mistake or even a near-miss, instead of starting an investigation with the attitude that someone has to be responsible and take punishment, we break it into two distinctly different systems. The most important one is the accident and incident investigation function, which we've learned how to do by studying the National Transportation Safety Board's methods. That gives us the facts to use in deciding what the contributing factors were, and then to immediately go after the urgent job of correcting each of those identified systemic contributors. Recall I made a point of the fact that there is never a root cause, but always root causes, plural? But once that investigative function is complete, we then look at the event to see whether instead of just human mistakes, we might be dealing with a failure to rise to the level of professional conduct we expect, including whether our rules were violated.

"Only when we have all the facts in front of us can we ask that question, and if the answer is 'No,' that's the end of it, and we'll fight tooth-and-tong any state agency that wants to go after our guy or gal's license. But if it comes up as a 'Yes' — in other words if it appears that there was a breach of professional responsibility in some form and not just a human mistake — then we shift to an entirely different mode. We've adopted the attitude United Airlines is credited with helping to pioneer, a philosophy that we don't hire amateurs, and therefore if one of our professionals fails to rise to the professional standards expected of him or her, we need to repair the situation and get that person back in the saddle. Of course, if we're dealing with a purposeful act or something heinous, that dictates its own conclusion. But even when someone truly falls beneath the standards we expect of them, then our prime concern is how to correct future performance. Purely reactive punishment accomplishes nothing. Our approach is to see if retraining, perhaps additional education, or in the case of an addiction, a stringent rehab program, will solve the problem. But our attitude is we want you back and working and happy if at all possible and reasonable."

"Sometimes it's just a horrible mistake by a team and everyone's devastated, but no one's a bad actor."

"Absolutely. One of the people we've had help us recommends three stages of approaching this. The first where there's no real breach of procedures or methods, you just console. The second, you coach. The third, you fire. I personally think that's too simplistic, but it embodies the right stair-stepped idea."

"Jack, I'm aware of that huge change at United back in the '90s. I assume you've heard the tale of the 747 that almost hit the San Bruno Hill on takeoff from San Francisco?"

"No, I must have missed that one. Tell me."

"Do we have time for the story?"

"Sure. Alice Quinn is supposed to come get you in my office when she's ready."

"Okay, I'll keep it brief, but this one really impressed me. The basics are these: A full load of nearly 400 passengers headed for Hong Kong in a Boeing 747-400 model. The morning fog layer starts at 50 feet above the runway, there's a relief captain and copilot in the cockpit along with the flight captain and copilot, and as soon as the cockpit rises into this pea-soup fog and the wheels leave the ground, the outboard engine on the right wing begins compressor stalling — a gigantic series of surges and bangs that shakes the cockpit so profoundly that the crew can't even read the instruments. It's the copilot's leg, and he's flying on instruments, of course, and the captain is so rattled he fails to take control. As they're trying to deal with this incredibly distracting emergency, the relief copilot suddenly realizes that their heading has drifted almost 30 degrees to the right, and they're aimed directly at the San Bruno Hill, which is covered with antennas and fog. He yells for them to 'Pull up!' and the copilot yanks on the yoke so hard the relief captain now yells that they're going to stall if they don't push the nose down. The banging and shaking is still going on, and by the time they get it all under control and get the engine shut down, they've missed hitting the hill in the fog by about 50 feet. Jack, that's 750,000 pounds of people, bags, and fuel barely missing the top of the hill by about one-sixth the length of the fuselage."

"Yikes!"

"The FAA departure controllers are aware there is an emergency, but they don't realize the flight has almost crashed. They vector the pilots around for a landing, and when the airplane is parked at the gate, the effects of United's new philosophy kicks in. Now, that's the same thing you're teaching here, but before the mid-'90s, any United pilots reporting that they'd so mishandled an emergency that they almost killed everyone on board would have probably been suspended or fired, and certainly considered weak sisters. But United had broken with tradition and realized that getting good information on near misses was far more important than just exercising their power and firing someone. They adopted the philosophy that 'We hire professionals, and if professionals fail, the first question for the system is, how did we help them fail?' United, in effect, told their pilots, 'If you screw up and it wasn't purposeful and you report it promptly, we'll self-disclose to the FAA and protect you from any professional sanctions.' Now, imagine that scene, Jack. Here are these four highly professional and experienced pilots sitting totally adrenalized in this parked cockpit, and in previous years they would have concluded a pact to say nothing. Sound familiar?"

"What, Will," Jack snorted, "Do you think an OR full of doctors would ever do that?"

"No, of course not. Anyway, with these pilots, instead of a pact of silence and denial, all four of them 'beat feet' to the chief pilot to tell the entire tale. True to their promise, United starts looking into the details instead of going for their throats. They assume there must be a systemic problem, and there was a doozy of a problem. It turns out that these four pilots — and every other 747 pilot in the world — had been improperly trained by simulators that were not programmed to simulate what actually happens in that kind of takeoff power compressor stall. In other words, this crew had been totally unprepared because the training system had failed them, and only because of United's changed cultural attitude were United and all 747 operators able to fix the problem in time."

A steady stream of people had been flowing around Jack and Will as if they were a well-known rock in a stream, and Jack now took the younger physician's elbow and pointed down the corridor.

"Let's go to my office and get out of everyone's way, Will.

Besides, I've got something to show you on my desk."

Jack preceded him into his office and fumbled around with something on the credenza behind his desk before turning around and slapping at something gold on his left lapel. Whatever the device was, it responded to his slap with a series of electronic chirps, and Will realized the CEO was grinning at him.

"What is that?" Will asked, smiling cautiously.

"That's my genuine, official, Star Fleet lapel communicator."

"Uh, huh. So, you don't just use *Star Trek* as an example, I'm dealing with a full-blown Trekkie."

Jack pulled the magnetically attached pin from his lapel looking a bit sheepish. "Well, not really a Trekkie, although I do drop by that exhibit in Vegas every time I'm there because the mockup of the bridge on the Enterprise is awesome. The reason I talk about that show, Will, is what it tells us about commandership versus leadership."

Jack plopped down in one of the two chairs on the other side of his desk and regarded Will over the small coffee table.

"Do you know the show at all? Either the original version in the '60s or the one 20 years later called *The Next Generation*?"

Will chuckled. "Yeah, I do. Not intimately so that I could tell you what happened in each episode..."

"Well, I can't do that either, but I can tell you that both of us were trained to be Captain Kirk, and Captain Kirk is deadly."

"How do you mean?"

"As a physician, not a CEO, what are you supposed to be, Will? Leader or commander?"

He thought for a second before looking back at Jack. "Well, both, I'd guess."

"Okay, let me define my terms, as Voltaire used to counsel. A commander is omnipotent and infallible and must know his job and the jobs of everyone under his command. A commander needs no advice, just facts, and is always ready to bark orders at whomever needs the direction. A commander should be intolerant of failure, especially in himself. A *leader*, however, gauges himself or herself by how well that leader can extract, orchestrate and utilize all the human talent available to that leader. There are times when a leader has to operate as a commander, such as when directing a code, but most of the time a true, effective leader leads by listening, and gathering and filtering information and advice, as well as facts, in order to make superior decisions. A leader never forgets that human infallibility is impossible. Got it?"

"I think so. With those definitions, I'd say doctors are trained to be commanders, not leaders."

"You got it."

"And, Jack, I think most hospital CEOs tend to be leaders more often than commanders."

"Well, mostly right, with exceptions. Sets up an interesting dynamic, doesn't it, when you think about commander-oriented doctors dealing with leader-oriented hospital CEOs who aren't docs?"

"These are ideas I'd never considered."

"Let me get back to Jim Kirk. Captain James Tiberius Kirk, to be exact, was played by William Shatner, the actor who had so much fun on that show *Boston Legal*. What Shatner and the writers of the original *Star Trek* got absolutely right about the captain was his attitude toward commandership, that air of omnipotence and that urgent need to be right each and every time."

"As I recall the character of Kirk, he was a bit cartoonish."

"At times, yeah. He was always looking for an opportunity to rip his shirt off and fight something, or chase some female to another planet. But other than that silliness, Kirk was extremely typical of the paradigm. One senior Air Force officer friend of mine told me that as he entered pilot training, he was advised to watch reruns of *Star Trek* and study Kirk so he'd know how a really good commander conducted himself. But 20 years later, a new crop of Hollywood writers gave us a captain that was representative of an entirely new form of command-leadership, the same sort of individual the airlines were trying to create."

"You're talking about *Star Trek: The Next Generation*?"

"Absolutely, and the new captain, Jean-Luc Picard. When they started promoting the new show I was excited. I thought, this is great, we're going to get a new Kirk, but then I watched a few episodes and wondered what the devil they were thinking by putting this weak guy Picard in command of the new starship. I mean, when something went wrong on his ship, Kirk would barrel up to the bridge, bark out incredibly wise and clever orders, and save the day. But when something threatened Picard's crew and ship, instead of barking orders and knowing exactly what to do, he'd call a freaking staff meeting! I remember thinking, *What a wuss.* He'd gather his senior officers around a table and ask their professional opinion. As a med student I remember being warned that to ask someone else's opinion, especially in front of a patient, would seriously undermine my image and trustworthiness as a doctor. Well, here's Captain Picard *asking*, and I thought, they're going to run all over him. But as the months and the episodes unfolded, I realized what the writers were doing. This commander wasn't weak at all. He was as strong and sure and effective as any human could be, but he was a far better leader because he admitted to being an imperfect human who didn't always have the right answer. In fact, he took real pride in his leadership ability to get the best out of his crew because he knew that what they could do together no human captain could achieve alone. I've never seen a piece of popular culture highlight the difference between commandership and leadership as well as the contrast between the two *Star Trek* captains. Since we were all trained to be Kirk — doctors, airline pilots, military professionals — the distinction is absolutely vital."

"Who was your favorite character, Jack? Spock?"

"Definitely not. Mr. Spock was a walking computer. No, my favorite was the guy we saw about 40 minutes into each episode standing at the view screen in the engine room and looking upset. In the background there was always smoke and steam. The dilithium crystals were melting down, they were moments away from imploding, and at least two bodies were on the floor — both clad in the red uniform shirts that signaled at the start of the hour that they were going to die — and this fellow says in a thick Scottish accent, 'Captain, we're givin' ya as much power as she's got down here. The engines canna take much more!'"

"Scotty!"

"Yep. Got to meet him once... at least the actor, Jim Doohan. I liked his character best because he was the model of the type of copilot or engineer the airlines have now created. Scotty was the perfect nurse or receptionist or resident. He was respectful, strong, professional, and he was never, ever reluctant to speak up when something needed to be passed — even when Kirk clearly did not want to hear it."

Will was nodding energetically. "That willingness to speak up by subordinates is the crux of the CRM courses they teach to airline crews — crew resource management."

"Yes. Although, I think we're light years beyond those basic lessons with the way we approach inter-team communication here at St. Michael's. But the principles of CRM were the starting point for the massive cultural changes in aviation, and Tenerife was the starting point for CRM. The leader is required to lead with full participation of his crew, the crew is required to be assertive with respect, and the leadership of the overall system is required to be 100 percent supportive in sanctioning or firing a captain who refuses to adopt the method."

"Much easier in aviation, of course, where everyone works for the same entity, which is why you've unified everyone here with those agreements covering the medical staff."

"Right, but I'll let you in on a secret, Will. It's something a number of startled airline chief pilots found out after worrying that they'd have to fire a quarter of their senior captains for refusing to adopt CRM. When we first started instituting all these seismic changes, even with most of our physicians on board and actively participating in designing the new procedures and protocols, we had a few very senior guys whose attitude was that they could not and would not be dictated to. The more we tried to get them into the process, the more they resisted, and worse, the more they tried to start a stampede in the opposite direction. So, we had to shoot a couple of the leaders to turn the herd."

"You what?"

Jack sighed at the memory, and seconds passed before he continued.

"I had to let go two of my best surgeons. It was a very tough decision because both of these fellows were very fine people, but they were destroying our efforts. They were both absolutely flabbergasted. Neither of them expected I'd be so tough, and each ran out and lawyered up and threatened legal mayhem, and I just stood my ground. The prediction from some of my key people was that my actions would unravel everything and cause a sympathetic exodus of many other physicians. Instead, some of the other physicians who had been almost as bellicose started quieting down, and within a few weeks the message could be heard rumbling around the physicians' lounge that if we were that damned determined, maybe it was worth a try.

"My biggest pushback after that was from a nervous board that went very white when I told them we were going to lose the considerable revenue these two dismissed gentlemen brought in. In fact, the hardest part was trying to convince the board that these two big surgeons leaving wasn't the threat, it was what would happen if we let them stay and destroy our patient safety program. They were very nervous, but they'd pledged to back me and they did, and I told them we'd survive it and we did. The airlines had the same experience. Once the majority of the dissenting captains realized their company was dead serious about dismissing those who wouldn't conform — once just two or three captains were cashiered — the rest fell into line with remarkable speed because they really didn't want to have the same experience. Same thing here."

"Painful though, right?"

"The magnitude of the change we were attempting involved so many lives and so much money, Will, I didn't have the option of being conciliatory or compromising. You'll find you'll have to be equally as hard-nosed if you lead such a change." Jack glanced at his watch. "I'm expecting Alice to show up in scrubs any minute and haul you off to the OR, but until she shows, one more thing I didn't discuss yesterday. We used to think there were two basic aspects to an effective safety system in medicine. The first is the process of trying to minimize human error through education, learning from previous accidents and incidents, instilling forcing functions, and doing anything else we can do to keep the errors from occurring in the first place. But we know the errors are still going to happen, and we can predict what they'll be. So the second part is designing our system, and our attitudes, to not only *expect* errors but be fully ready to catch them and safely absorb them long before they can affect a patient."

"You have a pet example?"

"Bunches of them. For instance, we know that regardless of how careful our nurses are, at some point in time a nurse is going to approach a patient with a lethal dose of something even though she is absolutely convinced it's the right medication, right dose, right path. If we know this, and we do, then we build a final prophylactic buffer into the system by using bar-coding at the bedside as the last, best chance to safely absorb that error. Or, if we can't afford the machinery, we require a final check, or maybe — if we can postulate the luxury of hiring enough nurses — we require a second nurse to double-check the medication before it's administered. The point is, we know the error will still occur despite best efforts, so we prepare to deflect it."

"Okay. Step one, prevent. Step two, anticipate and deflect."

"Right, but we now know we were missing a major third step."

"The see-saw principle. Janice explained it to me."

"Well, it's an incredibly important discovery, and it goes to the heart of our method. If we *ever* get to assuming we have it all handled and anticipated and protected, that's precisely when our well-trained team will decide that some small indication of trouble couldn't be right, and no one will speak up. Or, worse, someone speaks up and there's a quick assurance that hey, don't worry, it really is at 15, 15, green."

"Or, Jack, in your example, the nurse is unknowingly carrying that lethal dose of the wrong stuff, there is no other nurse to help her catch it, the bar-coding reader is broken or missing, or she's become used to bypassing it, and anyway she's pressed for time and in her heart-of-hearts she knows there's really no problem because she's certain the dose is correct."

"That's right. Without the see-saw principle, she'll inject the dose and kill the patient. With it, the nurse — albeit grudgingly — has to assume the dose is potentially lethal and therefore she is professionally constrained to take another close look at it in accordance with the agreed procedure."

"And she thereby catches the error at the last possible moment, right?"

"Right. Provided she faithfully follows the procedure, which requires constant reinforcement, peer pressure, and constant retraining, all of which will be required until the culture completely changes to embrace the same paradigm. Remember Dr. James Reason, Will?"

"The British researcher? Yes, I've read at least one of his books and heard him cited endlessly."

"With good reason. He's the man who gave us the Swiss Cheese Model, in which each of the defense methods standing against any systemic catastrophe are stylized as slices of Swiss cheese. Each defense method has holes and exceptions through which an error can pass, so individually, each defense slice is flawed. But if you put enough of the flawed slices together, the holes won't line up. If a potentially lethal error can't find a tunnel all the way through the stack, if the error is stopped by just one of a half-dozen or a dozen defense slices regardless of their individual imperfections, the error can't reach the patient. The idea is not that each defense method, or slice of cheese, is perfect and unfailing and without holes, it's that enough of these flawed slices put together essentially cancel out one another's incapacities and become an effectively impenetrable shield. So we build backups to back up the backup systems backing up the backups, and despite the fact that each backup system or method is imperfect, together they lower the potential for a patient injury to nearly zero. Same principle Boeing uses to build jetliners with enough backup systems to handle any reasonably anticipatable series of failures. Same method we've used to bar terrorists from commercial airline cockpits. And it's how we're keeping our patients safe at last."

"So," Will countered, "the system can accommodate someone taking a shortcut and still work."

"No! Absolutely not. See, that's a key point, Will. If we effectively create an air-tight system against medical error with, say 21 steps and procedures and protocols, and it works, it very well may work because we have 21 barriers versus 20. In other words, take only one barrier away — stop using the see-saw principle or negative assumption with medications, for instance, and we may find it was that 21st step that saved the lives of a dozen patients. No, that's why standardization is so important, and why no one can be allowed to deviate from an established series of prophylactic methods that together have been proven effective."

"Jack, I have a friend who ran a very large hospital until this past year, and he was an absolute dynamo on patient safety. I know he didn't achieve the atmosphere you've created here, but he was running a far larger hospital in a major western city with a board that supposedly gave him carte blanche to improve safety performance. And he really created very interactive teams. He kept telling his board that while some changes were already working, the majority of the cultural change would take at least a decade, but all they could see were dollar signs, and when he couldn't produce enough cost savings directly related to all the patient safety advances, they violated their promises and fired him. I mean, how can we ever expect to achieve all these things you've done here if the average board is too scared to follow through and understand how long it takes to change a culture with so much inertia?"

"You can lead a horse to water, Will..."

"I know, but it's depressing."

"Here's the deal. We know what works and how to make it work. We now know how to protect patients as well as the staff and the hospital itself. We know, as well, that to uphold the public trust we have no ethical choice. But are we willing to spend the money and take the risks and stay the course in order to do what's right and, what will be ultimately the most profitable even for non-profits? I have my board's assurances and promises and so far they've been strong and honest about those commitments. But could I see a revolt in the future because they panic over money? Yes, they could get scared and lose sight of their public trust as well as the reality that culture change takes at least a decade. They could lose faith in me and start listening instead to some panicked finance guy who doesn't believe in anything he can't quantify. But that's the risk I take. That's the risk your friend took. We can cajole and teach and lead, but ultimately it's the board members of hospitals across America that will either make hospitals into high-reliability institutions, or will thwart improvements to the point that we all end up nationalized and run by some giant bureaucracy in Washington. Sorry to interject a downer, but it's a fact we have to face. There are hundreds of CEOs out there who won't even try to risk change, unless ordered to do so, because they're myopically focused on the bottom line and running scared."

"These are good people who, along with their boards, have been dragged down by fear of financial failure."

"That's right. They're like a sea captain who's left his bridge to race around the ship personally directing preparations for a storm while the ship is steaming full speed toward a reef. They get to the point of fearing financial trouble more than patient deaths and injuries, and they become terribly shortsighted. These are the well-intentioned guys and gals who wear you down demanding financial justification and cost-benefit proof on every idea and every program until the patient safety people just give up. They submerge into micromanaging everything and every dollar and lose sight — if they ever had it — of the vision, and substitute misguided faith that tactical methods and incremental changes in procedures will do the job. I tell you, Will, if their attitude prevails, ultimately they'll sink us as an American institution."

"What you're talking about, Jack," Will said, his eyes lighting up, "is a concept I encountered in my MBA program called 'knowledge utilization.'"

"I've heard of it, but I'm not schooled in it."

"It's a method of systematically structuring who should deal with the various types of information and knowledge coming into a system or a company. In other words, it asks, 'What information do people need to do their best job in the positions they hold?' In nautical terms, the captains need the strategies and the tactics, but the admirals — as you just said — are the ones the organization absolutely depends on to hold tight to the vision and keep them on course. You can't do that if you're down in the weeds all the time doing the job of the captains."

"Or getting in the way of the captains," Jack added, nodding vigorously and sitting forward. "Will, I know that discipline by a slightly different route. Remember CRM, crew resource management? Part of the discipline is a cockpit version of what you just said. If, in an airliner cockpit something goes wrong, the captain needs to assign tasks to the appropriate people while he or she maintains the overall control of the situation and keeps them moving in the right direction."

"You're identifying something else I really didn't do right when I was trying to run my hospital."

"Micromanaging?"

"Yes, although I don't think I ever lost sight of the vision."

"You can't use that word without defining it carefully, Will. By some definitions, my cheerleading and cajoling everyone to keep us on course toward the vision is considered micromanaging. But while I don't get in the way of my captains, my nurse-managers or directors or chiefs, I do empower them and I share governance with them. Otherwise I'd be the ascetic guru making disconnected pronouncements about vision from the top of a mountain no one visits."

"Understood. But, Jack, how do you sit a board member or a disbelieving CEO down and convince him that he's got to lead this cultural change, not just for patient safety, but for the basics of good medicine and in order to be responsive to the patient? It seems so many just think we're over the top with what I was trying to do at my former hospital and what you've actually accomplished at St. Michael's. How do you convince them there's no other rational, ethical, moral or financially stable course?"

"Let me try this, Will. In 1999 when the IOM threw its bomb, we could only guess at what would truly work to drastically reduce patient injuries, deaths and near misses. People could argue against moving too fast because we really weren't sure. Now we are. Now we know what works and what doesn't work, and it's deceptively simple. Hospitals that decide to change themselves have a template on what steps to take, and we're one of the living laboratories. It's not painless, it's not cost-free, and it's nothing short of a decade-long cultural revolution. But it works. True, the resultant cost savings will take time to actually show up and be provable, but as long as the changes can be made without financial collapse, and they can, then you have to ask yourself as a CEO or a board member: 'Am I violating the public trust if my hospital doesn't do what St. Michael's is doing down in Denver?' And I would answer that with a resounding 'Yes!' To stop short of our level of commitment is a violation of public trust, and we will all pay a heavy price if those attitudes don't change."

"Jack, in my case, I thought I'd changed my hospital, and after several years we had a terrible tragedy." Will felt his voice catch and fought for control. "I..."

"Wait," Jack interrupted, "you've already told me you had a collection of parts, but not the whole. St. Michael's may yet commit a terrible mistake and create a human tragedy here, too, despite all our best efforts. But if that happens, we're not going to abandon everything. We'll still carry on with the program and try even harder and smarter, because we know our method works."

"Bonding people together, creating collegiality and expecting mistakes you can't fully eliminate?"

"Changing the sinew of the culture to work almost selflessly at times for the patient. The vision is really that simple." Jack sighed, his eyes drifting to something on an upper level of his office bookcase. "Boards of directors or trustees like the ones that panicked and fired your friend are defeating themselves and running from their responsibilities. Their hospital will never change without his type of dedicated pressure and leadership. Your buddy was a pacesetting leader who began major cultural changes but hadn't had the decade necessary to inculcate them, right?"

"Essentially, yes."

"Well, they made a huge, if not fatal, mistake. And so do boards that overreact to a tragedy after years of patient safety improvement with the idea that all that money and effort has been wasted. It's hard to navigate a ship through a storm without wanting to panic and reverse course, but turning around is often the most dangerous thing to do. You've safely sailed past the worst of the rocks and the reefs and now you're going to have another go at it? It's not cowardice as much as panic. Throwing out a driving force, a good leader, in the middle of a culture-changing campaign sets back the entire institution and leaves patients much less safe."

"Yeah, well, in my case, I resigned because I felt I'd failed. They didn't force me out."

"But they didn't exhort you to stay and fight on either, did they?"

"No, they didn't. Of course, I had none of the great solutions you've incorporated here."

"You had determination, and that's a large part of the battle of leadership in cultural change. But we're a David battling the Goliath of mindless inertia, 'the way we've always done it' syndrome. Tell me this isn't cost effective immediately — everything we're doing — and I'll tell you you're probably right. But I'll also tell you that to fail to energetically follow our lead when we know what works is to doom some of your patients every year to death, and more to life-altering injuries, and that's a de facto violation of everything a hospital ought to stand for. If you want to sail in a boat that floats and I tell you that, to do so, you need to repair the holes in the hull and not just be exceptional at bailing, it would be pretty stupid of you to go sailing off without plugging those holes, right? Well, that's the same principle. Want to keep your patients safe and satisfied? Here are the ways to accomplish that, how to make a high-reliability organization out of a high-risk enterprise. You want that result B? Then you use method A. That simple. But if you think it's okay to keep on killing a few hundred thousand patients a year and feeding the coffers of malpractice lawyers because change is deemed too expensive or too difficult, or too scary and uncertain, then go ahead and avoid change and keep on doing it the same way. Maybe you'll retire before it all comes to grief. But the piper will be paid. Eventually, if we don't change this system, Congress will end up taking control to mollify an outraged electorate, and none of us will like the results."

Jack was getting to his feet and nodding toward the door. "And here is our surgical chief ready to show you her cockpit... ah, I mean... OR."

"Funny, Jack," a pleasant female voice said from behind as Will stood and took her offered handshake. She rolled her eyes in Jack's direction. "Our CEO, who uses too many nautical metaphors and would make this office into a replica of a ship's bridge if he could, likes to needle me for borrowing so much from cockpit procedures."

"She thinks she's a pilot, Will," Jack laughed.

"I *am* a pilot," she replied, "but I fly, you know, smaller stuff than airliners. Nevertheless, the principles are the same, as I'm about to show you. Follow me, Dr. Jenkins, and be careful not to trip over Jack's soapbox on the way out."

Will's Notes:

- Like it or not, I have to admit the Star Trek analogy is very apropos, especially in regard to contrasting commandership (Kirk) with true leadership (Picard).

- Best definition I've ever heard of leadership: "A leader measures himself or herself by how well that leader extracts, orchestrates and utilizes all the human talent available to that leader." Definition of a Commander: One who knows all, sees all, needs no help, and is both omnipotent and infallible — which is, of course, impossible.

CHAPTER ELEVEN

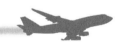

"Will, I had to fight hard to get into a surgical residency," Dr. Alice Quinn was saying as she kept up a brisk pace toward the surgical suites. "I was determined because I'd always wanted to be a general surgeon. I was well aware specialization was considered the best financial move, but I wanted to do as many different types of surgery as I could, and it's been that experience over the years as a general surgeon that laid the foundation for my own awakening."

"About patient safety, you mean?"

"Well, let me just say that if I hadn't personally committed just about all the patient safety sins there are, such as losing track of surgeries, patients, and procedures, if I hadn't literally fallen asleep with my hands in a patient one night after 30 hours with no sleep, I wouldn't have been able to shed the professional tunnel vision so easily and see how absurd we can be defending the way we've traditionally done things." She pointed to a wide corridor branching to the left. "We go this way."

Will stayed in lockstep with her as he gestured behind them as if the thought she'd just expressed had been left in the middle of the corridor.

"What do you mean by absurd?"

"Here we are," she said, stopping in front of a set of double doors, turning, and glancing down momentarily as if to order her reply, then meeting his eyes.

"We're a profession in denial. We've been like a raging alcoholic refusing to admit to a drinking problem. We've been contributing to, no, *creating*, major patient safety hazards with our lone-eagle attitudes and our extreme resistance to change."

"I couldn't agree more, Alice."

"We've acted like there's some deep, dark mystery to the procedures setting up and surrounding surgery, like we're a priesthood forming the only repository of the true faith of the practice. We act like there's a truth no one else is allowed to glimpse, when in fact the vast majority of even the most delicate surgeries are just what we call them, *procedures*! Each one has a beginning, a middle, and an end, just like a flight, and a lot of the ancillary stuff we can and should do the same every time, just like in aviation. By the way, did you know that the Anesthesia Patient Safety Foundation (APSF) hatched that comparison with aviation in the '80s, and most anesthesiologists know it well?"

"Comparing a surgery to a flight?"

"Specifically comparing a general anesthesia sequence to a flight. Takeoff, cruise, landing. *They* figured it out, but the attending surgeon at their side still too often thinks he or she doesn't need checklists, time-outs, standardized OR setups and safety protocols, even when overwhelming data exists to prove we do. What's worse, many of the attendings who have, shall we say, somewhat discounted the APSF's successes would be astounded to know that on average anesthesia performs with an error rate of five-sigma!" She motioned him over to a set of chairs. "We've actually got about 10 minutes. Let's sit out here a minute and talk."

He followed her and settled into one of the offered chairs.

"You, Will Jenkins," she smiled, "were looking skeptical a minute ago, and that's an expression I've grown very familiar with while ramrodding the cultural upheaval around here."

"Well, I guess I am a little bit. What I was going to say, Alice, is an obvious demurrer. A good surgeon is not just a technician, even in orthopedics, where I'll readily admit some of the procedures seem very mechanical. A good surgeon has a sixth-sense, a delicate, sometimes impossible-to-define instinct that couples with fine motor skills and steady judgment, and you can't create that with a checklist."

She was smiling as she came forward in the chair, an index finger raised for emphasis and her eyes sparkling. "You're right and you're wrong. You're right that you can't *create* such delicate, subjective skills with checklists and regimentation. But you're wrong if you're contending that you can't improve the ability to utilize those skills by minimizing variables and standardizing setups. Unfortunately, the very observation you just made — that same demurrer — has been used for decades by surgeons as a shield against change or any form of standardization in the OR. It's the, 'Surgery is magic and you can't regiment it' school of thought, and it's a dangerous smokescreen. Yes, without a doubt it's the surgeon's fine touch, nerve, experience, instinct, and feel that's so valuable, and those skills are not paint-by-the-numbers functions. But, the basic sequence of actions in an open heart procedure, for instance, *can* be ordered, standardized, and followed, and in fact *must* be if the procedure is going to be performed in accordance with best practices. Maverick actions such as stopping the heart too early before starting the process of connecting the patient to the heart-lung machine are not going to have a good result, right?"

"Obviously."

"Well, in any surgical procedure there are a myriad of things that can and should be done the same way every time, and by standardizing your approach to those items, you reduce the number of things a team has to worry about. More importantly, standardization reduces the extent to which your unconscious patient is forced to gamble that you're not going to make a mistake."

"By standardization, you mean steps such as assuring that it's the right patient on the table and the right medications standing by for injection and a thousand other things that are finite and necessary?"

"Well, I mean setting up the room the same way every time for a specific procedure, regardless of who the attending is. No preference cards, in other words. No unnecessary variability. The team members positioned the same for the same procedure, and using the very same precautionary procedures such as pre-surgical time-outs and specific protocols for making certain we've got the right patient, right site, right medications, and right paperwork and labs. It means a universal willingness, especially on the part of the surgeon, to cancel the surgery in a heartbeat, and without rancor, if *everything* doesn't line up."

"Rather like the willingness of a pilot to break off an approach and go around if things are not looking right?"

"Absolutely! Traditionally we've been terrible at that, getting angry, lashing out at whoever we think the 'guilty' party is who didn't finish the paperwork, and too often acting like petulant children, all of which disciplines the team into never challenging anything. That's why one of the steps I instituted here focuses on teaching our docs to compliment and reward surgical team members who catch a problem and cause a surgery to be canceled, even if their mistake caused the problem to begin with. Our focus, after all, is not to demonstrate how perfect our people can be. Our purpose is to do the best job for the patient, and that means having an instantaneous willingness to stop things when we're not absolutely sure we're ready, checked and safe."

"I've studied the use of checklists, but all the docs in my former facility were uncomfortable with them."

"Let me guess, the 'cookbook medicine' complaint, right?"

"Among others."

"What they have to be taught, and they won't practice here if they don't accept, is that the checklists and the protocols for safety are not there to order or direct the fine art of a surgeon's abilities, they're there to minimize the chances every patient takes with a surgical procedure while leaving we surgeons free to concentrate on what we do best. As I said before, and this is kind of a buzz phrase around here, our patients do not agree to let us gamble with their lives just to demonstrate how good we are at doing things our own way. And that's what ignoring standardization and best practices really constitutes — unwarranted gambling."

"How far do you take the push for standardization? Everything the Joint Commission or IHI says, for instance?"

"No. We adopt nothing without hammering out a professional consensus on what should be standardized, and even then, sometimes, it's startling the areas we hadn't thought about. Let me give you a rather funny example. A few months ago our orthopedics nurse-manager sat down one evening and made out a chart to reflect the various post-surgical dressing requirements of the 16 surgeons whose patients flowed onto her floor. There were 26 basic dressing requirements covering six basic types of surgeries, from knee and hip replacement to back surgeries. While there was some duplication, essentially every surgeon demanded different dressing requirements in each category. Multiply 26 times 16 and you get 416 separate dressing requirements for 16 surgeons. The result, in other words, required either a massive checklist for her 70 nurses, or a substantial change. So one day she asks to speak to the orthopods in their grand rounds, and manages to coax all 16 into being there. It's 7 a.m. and she opens with what she calls a brief PowerPoint presentation, explaining that she wants to make absolutely sure she is putting out the correct requirements for her nurses to follow. 'Now,' she says, 'we use one inch sterri-strips to reinforce our hip incisions. That is, except for Dr. White, who likes the sterri-strips cut in half. And… Dr. Wilson, who wants betadine applied first.' She catalogues the different dressing preferences of each doctor then moves on to the next slide, which lists all the different mobility precautions — for the same surgery — by physician. By the time she gets to the third slide, which lists the different hematocrit levels by physician as to when additional blood is needed, they're all shifting in embarrassment in their chairs. Finally, one of the doctors raises a hand. 'Okay!' he says, all but hiding his face. 'Okay, Kathleen. We get the picture.' The orthopedic docs then and there forged an agreement to meet and hammer out a method of agreeing to single-method dressings in each category, eventually dropping from some 416 separate variations to fewer than 30. *That's* the sort of grassroots cooperative change we've sparked here, but as I say, it's sometimes staggering how many areas we overlook because that's the way it's always been done."

"That's a heck of an example! But they agreed to simplify?"

"They saw how ludicrous it was, thanks to the way the nurse-manager presented it."

"Impressive."

"There's one other important point I need to make, Will. Rather than interfere with a surgeon's skills, all the precautions we've put in place give our surgeons room to concentrate on the procedure itself without spending mental energy sweating the routine stuff or blindly depending on the others in the room to be perfect."

"There's no question good procedures prevent travesties such as operating on the wrong leg."

"Or the wrong patient," she replied, nodding. "Absolutely. And we do spend a lot of background energy worrying about making the 'big' mistake. We don't even talk about how devastating the psychological effect can be on physicians when someone gets badly hurt on their watch, or while under their knife. Consider the tragic impact of walking out of an OR knowing you've performed a brilliant double mastectomy and reconstructive technique on a young woman. Her reconstructed breasts will look close to normal, and you're proud of that, until you discover that she wasn't in for a mastectomy. She's the wrong patient, and you just impacted, if not devastated her life. If that's too clinical, imagine it was another surgeon doing the cutting and it was your beautiful young 20-year-old daughter on the table."

"Point well taken."

"By the way, we personalize such examples around here to keep our focus clear. They may be 'cases,' but our 'cases' have names and lives and we can't be cavalier about their humanity. This is how we preserve the integrity of our work."

"Believe me, I understand."

"That unnecessary mastectomy actually happened, Will, more than once around the country. One victim was even featured on *Good Morning America* in 2006. This is precisely the sort of risk we always run when we do things the way we've always done them. So, to put it bluntly, we've stopped gambling with our patients' welfare. We don't assume we're cutting the right patient, we make absolutely sure. We don't assume the scrub nurse is handing us a syringe with the right medication, we make absolutely sure. We do not have the right to take extra risks with our patients just to establish our autonomy as physicians. Our patients don't give us that authority."

"You know, I never really viewed a surgeon doing things his own way as gambling, but that's a powerful analogy."

"It's one thing if a tomcat of a pilot goes out flying a light airplane by himself over an unpopulated area and arrogantly disregards the best practices in aviation by refusing to use checklists or flight plans. It's an entirely different matter if he does it with trusting passengers aboard, or over populated terrain. Same principle. Your decision to take a known and excessive risk should never imperil others; In the OR we're not cutting on ourselves."

"How is the level of communication among your OR teams?"

"Superlative, if I do say so. We've either retrained or eliminated those who insisted on intimidating their surgical team members. Instead, we've trained our attendings to take pride in admitting they can't be perfect, and that therefore they need the help of everyone in the room."

"You're talking about the surgeon listening when someone speaks up?"

"Yes, but beyond that. We train our teams to verbalize even the most vague and unsupported feelings. Such as, 'Ah, Doc, I've got a funny feeling I read somewhere on the chart that this patient has a latex allergy. Could you hold on a second and let me check?' Now, can you imagine a young resident or a circulating nurse saying that in the traditional OR environment, especially with a grouchy attending? Here, the only acceptable response from the surgeon is, 'Absolutely, take a look; I'll wait.' And even if the nurse or the intern is dead wrong, that surgeon, after the procedure, is taught to take the time to put a supportive hand on the shoulder of that person and say: 'Good job! You might have been mistaken this time, but you could also have been right, and that is *exactly* what I want you to do! Thank you!'"

"So, you succeed in getting everyone to speak up, but, to play devil's advocate for a minute, what if you accidentally empower Attila-the-nurse who's never before had a voice and is now going to speak up at every opportunity to tell you how to practice? Way over the top, in other words, or even retaliatory for all the years of intimidation. How do you handle *that*?"

"Well, let me ask you this, Will. Are you in command if you're the attending in that scenario?"

"Yes."

"Then there's a price for being the leader. We expect you to be a teacher as well. It's *your* responsibility to take that person aside in a non-threatening, supportive way later and say, 'Look, let me help you with the proper way to exercise this responsibility to speak up.' Some people are naturals at this, and some suck at it, but for the latter category — surgeons who don't think it's their job and complain about lousy nurses — we don't have much patience. We make a concerted effort to retrain them, and then we let their team determine if we've been successful. If not, and the doc is resistant or cynical or just refuses to change and will not take responsibility for effectively training his team members, we give him the opportunity to choose another hospital, since his privileges end here."

"Just like that?"

"Hey, if he were scheduled to operate on your son and refused to follow our protocols, would you let him stay and do the procedure?"

"No, but that seems a bit harsh just because a surgeon isn't a good professor."

"You're missing the reason for us being so hard-nosed. Are you familiar with the 'halo effect?'"

"Yes. The tendency of subordinates to assume a superior couldn't be wrong because that senior individual has so much experience and position. We put kind of a halo over his head."

"Or her head. Yes, dead on. Well, here's the problem. Attending surgeons automatically have a halo above them in the eyes of many subordinate team members. In addition, few of us really know the full profile of how we come across in our verbal and facial expressions under stress. Even professional broadcasters or actors with decades of experience have to struggle at times to be sure they're coming across exactly as they intend in terms of facial expression, vocal timbre and apparent attitude. Now, take an attending who truly doesn't realize that when he corrects someone under a pressurized situation it sounds like a stinging rebuke. His eyebrows flare, his voice is sharp and perhaps sarcastic, and the recipient may feel badly assaulted, even though the attending didn't mean it that way. A nurse, for instance, may feel she's been slapped across the room and demeaned. But unless that nurse is trained to hold her ground and discuss it calmly with the attending later on, unless he or she has the courage and the unquestioned support of the hospital, that nurse will most likely just slink off in pain and lick her wounds, and in that case, two things happen, neither of them good. First, she'll eventually tell her closest friends and colleagues what happened, and resentment will spread against that attending. Second, the next time she's in an OR with that doctor, she'll be nervous, on guard, resentful and anything but a fully functioning member of the team. In other words, that one little snappy comment which the surgeon has long since forgotten has now trained this nurse to be distant and unresponsive and, above all else, very defensive. We had one doc last year who did exactly that and when a nurse manager asked him to sit down and discuss it, his response was: 'I hardly said anything to her! Your nurses need to develop thicker skins.'"

"And he's no longer here?"

"No, no! He's still here, but we guided him through a rather profound renaissance in understanding his critical role as leader and teacher and the fact that he has a responsibility to bite his tongue hard at times. We had to help him unlearn the essentially disrespectful and abusive ways *he* had been taught as an intern, and the way he'd seen arrogant senior professors treat nurses. He's a good guy. He got it. He even said, after he watched a video of himself barking at people in the OR, that he wouldn't have allowed someone like him to touch one of his kids."

"You seem to default to that analogy a lot — the family member as patient."

"Will, we use that comparison and analogy around here with impunity, especially when someone's being resistant or petulant. We teach professionals how to say, 'Excuse me, but would you make the same decision if that were your child on the table?' Amazing how even the most jaded of us can be stopped in mid-sentence."

"How are we doing on time, Alice?"

"Let's go inside."

They moved together into the pre-op area where Alice ran through the names of the surgical team they'd be observing. "They'll start their pre-brief in about five minutes," she said, her eyes suddenly wandering to a nurse who was drawing medications into syringes in a corner of the room. A second nurse had come through the door and was heading for the first one, apparently with a question. Will watched as Alice quickly stepped toward the entering nurse, a finger to her lips. The nurse's hands flew to her face in recognition as she smiled and mouthed the word "Sorry" before turning and leaving.

"What was that about?" Will asked when she'd walked back to him.

"We have a hard and fast rule that when someone's drawing up medication, no one interrupts, unless there's a code-level emergency or the building's on fire. It's so well inculcated in our habits now that all I had to do was gesture and Rachel knew precisely what I meant."

Will wrote a note to himself as she waited, then continued.

"Okay, the procedure we're going to watch, Will, is a total hip replacement, but the important thing is the way we prepare for it and carry out all the precautions we've instituted. I'd like you to do two things. First, observe all the steps that we do differently from other institutions, and second, please participate fully and give us the benefit of your professional critique on the debrief."

"You routinely do both a pre- and post-brief?"

"We require it, we do it, and we learn from every one of them. It doesn't take all that long provided there are no major complications. But there's something else you might not be prepared for, and we're really proud of our mutual decision to institute it."

"What's that?"

"We video every operation from six different camera angles."

"Video... *really*?"

"Really."

"So that's what you were referring to about the surgeon snapping at people — a video in the OR. And the medical staff went along with this?"

"They wrote the rules on when and how to use it. Of course we have very specific requirements for how the tapes can be used, all of which center around training and system improvement. No physician can be disciplined or sanctioned in any way based on one of the tapes, and even if something awful happens and a physician or nurse is professionally called on the carpet in a licensure matter, the tapes cannot be used and will not be produced."

"I would think you'd need a state law to protect them."

"That's what we're aiming for, but in the meantime, we have a hard policy that we will erase the tapes before we'll ever allow them to be used in a licensure case against one of our people. The exception would be a criminal case, when a tape could be considered protected evidence."

"And, on the subject of civil legal liability?"

"Hold onto your hat, Will. We've retained some very smart legal researchers who came back and validated what Jack and I both suspected, that the tapes are perhaps the best defense we could ever have against runaway liability."

"Okay, wait. How so? They're sure to get subpoenaed in any malpractice case."

"No one needs to subpoena them, we volunteer them."

"But why would you do that? A plaintiff's lawyer can twist anything around to work against you."

"In the extreme, yes. But consider this. _If_ our OR teams communicate the way we want them to, and _if_ they follow the protocols and procedures that we know work and are in the best interests of the patient, then the best evidence we could possibly produce that we performed as well as any human medical team could perform will be the HD quality video from six different angles, including all the readouts on the anesthesia machine. The very fact that we're willing to bring them forward voluntarily is a huge plus with a jury. Now, of course, if one of our docs or nurses comes completely unglued during a procedure and says or does something outrageous and unprofessional, the tapes would make it impossible for us to hide and lie. They keep any of us from ever getting caught trying to lie to a jury about what happened in a surgical procedure, but hiding things and trying to lie in court are the essential ingredients necessary to produce angry juries and mega-million dollar judgments."

She made a dismissive gesture. "But we have no business hiding or lying anyway, do we? You see, in effect, the tapes keep honest practitioners honest, and that's not only a good thing, that's the *only* ethical course of action. So, even if we make a mistake and an injury occurs, and the tapes provide an honest, if embarrassing, recitation of precisely what happened, they also provide invaluable guidance on how to change our system to prevent a repeat."

"But, when you give a tape up in a civil case, the state can get it to use in going after someone's license, right? Is that true here?"

"Yes, which is why we're pushing hard for a bill in the legislature to address just that problem by barring such use."

"I'm really shocked that you'd be brave enough to do this in the meantime."

"Well, that's part of the magnitude of the cultural overhaul. Plus, the legal risks are extremely minor compared to the benefits. You see the procedure as it unfolds, you hear the team members communicating constantly, you hear the attending talking everyone through the procedure and the anesthesiologist reporting as necessary, and even when something goes wrong, you witness a unified team of mutually respectful professionals working their hearts out to do the best possible job. So far, believe it or not, our lawyer thinks we've avoided at least three lawsuits with the tapes and our eagerness to provide them. More importantly, when we do lose a patient, our offer to show the entire sequence to a grieving family member is very reassuring, even if they never take us up on it."

"As I say, I'm rather astounded the physicians approved this. After all, we're a profession of paranoids, and for very good reason."

"But, Will, what are we doing in the OR that we want to hide?"

"Now, that's not the point."

"Yes, unfortunately, it is. Believe me we had plenty of our number react the same way. Taping in the OR? Not on your life! But we kept asking, what is it that you're worried about someone else seeing? Most replied that the legal liability scared them, and that lawyers twisted things, and juries would never understand what they saw and heard, and we countered those worries one by one, slowly and assuredly. In many respects those worries were as unrealistic as they were frightening. For others, the terrifying aspect was the chance that the media could get hold of a tape and misuse it to embarrass someone. HIPAA pretty much took care of that, though, since a medical procedure on tape is essentially a protected medical record. So at the end of the day, none of us could find any legitimate reason to oppose it, and once we started using it, the results were almost immediate. We've spotted and fixed process problems and communication problems we would have never known about, and our surgeons, me included, have actually changed the way we talk and inter-act as a direct result of hearing and seeing ourselves on those tapes." She chuckled. "It's amazing how you can sound so sure and authoritative in your own head and then find that the way you *really* came across was, well, a lot less impressive than you thought, especially when someone snaps at a team member. We replay something like that during the debrief, and no one has to make a negative comment. You vow right then and there to change your ways."

"Did you folks think that up here?"

"No. The airlines had the very same experience. They started videoing their simulator flights. A facilitator, or instructor, would attend the debrief and maybe point out to a captain that at a cer-tain point he had growled at, or demeaned, his copilot or refused to listen to a concern. All too often the captain would flatly deny it. 'I did no such thing! He misunderstood. *You* misunderstood!' So the instructor would play the tape back and the captain would sit there in the debriefing room with his mouth hanging open, and most were honest enough to say, 'I would have never believed it, but there I am doing exactly what you said I did.' The tapes were so powerful because they helped professionals correct themselves."

"So, all commercial cockpits are videoed?"

"Not in flight. Only the simulators. They don't tape in flight because their biggest pilot's union, ALPA, continues to oppose the idea of videotaping for analysis in the aftermath of an accident as well as the idea of videotaping for training and fine-tuning performance. They're dead set against it primarily because they don't trust the FAA or their employer airlines to do anything but use the tapes as a hammer with which to attack their members when any mistake is made. And frankly, neither the airlines nor the FAA have given them any reason for trust. For their part, the airlines are perfectly happy to have the taping blocked because taping would require special equipment and they don't want to spend an extra penny." She checked her watch. "Let's go, doctor. Pre-brief is set to start in two minutes and we've created a culture in there that does not like to start late."

Will's Notes:

Alice Quinn says the OR environment at St. M has been overhauled to incorporate the highest level of safety for the patient, which also helps provide the highest level of quality. The old way was to let surgeons do surgical procedures any way they professionally saw fit, as if they were individual artists and there was no justification scientifically or otherwise to force them to conform to anyone else's methods or procedures. She has a very important point. We've allowed surgeons to set up their ORs however they wanted and we gave them preference cards and harried nurses trying to conform to a different setup for every doctor. We've tolerated surgeons breezing in and starting an incision without so much as acknowledging the other members of the surgical team. We've let surgeons get comfortable over the years with never having a pre-brief or a post-brief on even the most difficult procedures, and for too long we let a few of them routinely get by with extreme behaviors such as throwing scalpels across the OR to demonstrate anger or disgust or frustration—almost a rule-by-terror in some cases. Generally, we conducted our surgeries and ourselves in such a bizarre and undisciplined, maverick way that the vast majority of our patents would have run in horror if they'd known the truth. Essentially our insistence on being so resistant to standardization has been putting our patients at risk, and that would have been a laughable concept a few years back.

Alice's recommendation for fixing it, and what they've done here:

First, admit that non-standardized surgical practice was an "absurd" way to do business insofar as providing reasonable levels of assurance that we've learned from past major mistakes and won't repeat the same tragedies, which is what standardization is all about. Second, change the attitude of the surgeon himself/herself. Bar-coded patients and wrist bands, and marking the right site and checking the charts are all important tactical measures, but the attitude of the attending toward the entire subject of standardizing and minimizing variables is primary.

Most surgeons are aware that the number of patients injured or killed across the nation from human errors is far too great to ignore. They all understand on at least some level that drastic change in old ways of practicing is coming whether they like it or not. But too many practitioners have dragged their feet and tried to ignore the problem as if it was someone else's challenge. On an individual basis, physicians still tend to cling to the lone-eagle approach—the idea that a doctor has to be totally independent, and that it is some sort of professional failure to ask for help. The thought patterns are self-abusive when you consider the inevitability of human mistakes, but regardless of what they say, physicians are trained to believe that if they concentrate hard enough and maintain a superlative level of vigilance and precision, they can avoid making the sort of terrible mistakes that befall lesser doctors. Of course, that attitude comes from the erroneous concept that good doctors don't make mistakes in the first place. Good doctors, therefore, will never need outside, not-invented-here procedures and protocols to protect against mistakes that we're not subject to making in the first place.

I always thought I was a good doctor, and now I know I am, but primarily because I admit to my inability to be perfect. That IS a hard stance to swallow, yet I know it's true.

What St. M has done is:

- Standardize procedures.

- Minimize variables.

- Outlaw preference cards for different surgeons when procedures can be standardized.

- Require full compliance with time-outs, both in spirit and execution, and both empower and require other OR team members to stop any surgical procedure if the established protocol is not followed (e.g., an attending tries to breeze past the time-out or pencil-whip it).

- Demand full communication among the team members, full participation, collegiality and consultation.

- No procedures without a substantive pre-brief and post-brief.

- Surgeons required to be really good and effective leaders vs. commanders.

- Surgeons held responsible and accountable for alienating team members or refusing to provide positive and sympathetic guidance to subordinates.

BIG POINTS:

Patients don't come to St. M to gamble, they come trusting their docs to help them.

Patients do NOT grant surgeons the right to gamble with their welfare just so a physician can demonstrate his autonomy.

BIG NOTE TO SELF: WHY IN THE WORLD AREN'T WE TEACHING THESE THINGS IN MEDICAL SCHOOL?

CHAPTER TWELVE

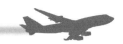

The spider-like pattern of stratospheric jet contrails laced a gossamer web high above Denver as Will alighted from the right seat of Jack's black H2 HUMMER and scanned the surrounding landscape. The steakhouse they'd chosen was in a far north suburb, and the prairies of northeastern Colorado were already showing the steep sun angles of late afternoon against the startling outlines of upscale housing developments, which sprouted like winter wheat in the distance.

"The area is obviously growing fast," Will commented, gesturing to the distant houses as Jack locked the huge vehicle and came around the front.

"Ridiculously so." He pointed to the north. "We expected Greeley and Loveland to kind of grow together with the overflow families streaming north from Denver and looking for nice homes, but these staccato developments are the way it looks almost all the way to the Wyoming border." He hesitated a second, smiling, as he gestured back over his shoulder. "So, you're not going to rag me about the HUMMER?"

"I figure just about everyone else at St. Michael's has already done that."

"Unmercifully. But to tell you the truth, I bought this monster just to compliment my image as an iconoclast. That, and I lend it to one of our scout troops all the time to haul kids around — safest thing short of a semi if they ever get into a wreck."

"Well, I'd say you deserve whatever the heck you want to drive, Jack," Will said as they headed into the restaurant. "After I left Alice, I went through the metrics you've generated for the last two years. I was already deeply impressed from what I read before I called you, but the staff satisfaction and patient satisfaction scores, the way you handle the safety reporting system and the drop in incidents, is just awe-inspiring."

Will pushed open the door of the restaurant and motioned Jack inside.

"It's not me, Will. It's a group thing, and that's not false modesty. Fact is, I've got great people. Without them, I'd be a lone cheerleader accomplishing nothing."

"Well, then you've done a heck of a job *finding* the right people."

"I'll take credit for some of the hiring, but most of the folks at St. Michael's, such as Alice, were already here. And I'll wager you that's the case all over the nation, hospitals filled with people of true talent and heart just waiting for someone to give them the support and the impetus to overhaul their culture."

The hostess escorted them to a booth and left them to study the menu. With a bottle of Australian Shiraz on the table and the meal ordered, Jack sat back with his glass and inclined his head in the general direction of his hospital with a knowing smile.

"So, Doctor, what did you think of our surgical arena? Details, now, not just accolades."

"Well, perhaps the best way I can put it is this. I've seen only two high-pressure environments run as well. One was a Boeing 777 cockpit, after an airline vice president worked for months to get me approved for a jump-seat ride, and the other was the control room of a nuclear power plant in Pennsylvania."

"How did they differ from the atmosphere in our OR?"

"Not by much. Professional, focused, quiet and completely communicative. Of course, the airlines and the nuclear power industry set the benchmarks for professional communication and checklist use. But the OR I experienced had pretty much the same feeling. It was just as Alice said, that the common interest everyone in that room shared was to do the best possible job for the patient, and that drove literally everything else. They ran the time-out with greater precision and professionalism than I've ever seen, with the attending leading the process, not just standing there looking disgusted, which is too often the response. The attending also talked everyone through the procedure, not excessively, but in such a way that we all knew precisely where he was in the process and what was coming next. The anesthesiologist was superb, too. Fully engaged, never looking bored or flipping through some magazine. He relayed in a quiet but steady stream of reports what was going on from his point of view so the attending was constantly updated. The nurses were in lockstep with the physicians, too, and they didn't hesitate to give them information, even as to an improperly positioned tray the scrub nurse had to deal with. The atmosphere in there, Jack, was neither tense, nor disengaged. We've experienced and heard about the extreme cases so often, but here it was just, well, amazingly comfortable. They worked as one."

"Did you hear much extraneous chatter? You know, about cars and vacations and the latest news?"

"No, now that you mention it. I think I recall a few quick references along the lines of, 'Looking forward to seeing you and your wife next week,' or 'Hope you enjoy that trip to Maui,' but other than that it was purely professional."

"Good."

"Is that because of the cameras and the recording?"

"No, it's because we borrowed something else from aviation that works incredibly well in principle. We all agreed that when the FAA imposed the 'sterile cockpit' rule on commercial aviation, they got it exactly right. And if airline cockpits should be sterile, or free of extraneous, non-pertinent and potentially distracting conversations during critical phases of takeoff, flight, and landing, then how can we justify not keeping the sterile field in an OR free of such chatter?"

"When did the FAA do that?"

"A long time ago, and during the administration of probably the worst FAA chief in history, but on this he was dead right. NTSB investigators had heard far too many accident sequences in which the cockpit voice recorder had captured excessive personal banter and extraneous chatter leading up to the actual accident. That was especially true for landing and takeoff accidents. Pilots would be so mentally wrapped up in a non-pertinent discussion that they were essentially flying the plane by rote, like a driver having a very serious conversation on a cell phone and concentrating so intensely that he loses track of the fact he's driving a car. So the FAA imposed a new rule, which was universally derided and ignored until the airlines themselves started enforcing it."

"But that's always the big difference, isn't it, Jack, between the airlines and our world? They can tell the pilots to do it or get fired, while we have to beg our physicians to please consider making a change."

"Yes and no is the answer to that. First, we don't beg our guys and gals here at St. Michael's because they themselves agree to those rules and the medical staff enforces them with real teeth, with us backing them completely. In other words, we do have the same degree of control as an airline: You'll do it the way we've all agreed to do it or you lose privileges and leave. But it's the second part of the equation that's the most fascinating, and I think the most relevant to us, and that's the silent, passive resistance. The philosophy behind the resistance to the sterile cockpit rule exhibited by airline pilots matches exactly the philosophy behind the resistance we, as doctors, have shown when faced with any attempt at regimenting our medical or surgical procedures."

"How is it similar to us? The FAA rule was a federal regulation that eventually got enforced."

"Yes, Will, but you had cockpits full of very bright pilots who thought the FAA was dead wrong and who were not about to let some flatlander bureaucrat tell them how to fly their airplanes. Oh, they grudgingly kept the personal conversations down about the time of takeoff or just before an instrument landing in bad weather, but for decades the resistance factor was so great that when accidents did occur, at least some extraneous conversations were still there on the cockpit voice recorder. Remember the 15, 15, green accident in Dallas? The voice tape was full of extraneous chatter, and that undoubtedly helped numb all three pilots to the point they were more vulnerable to totally misperceiving what the gauges said. Even the Comair crash in Lexington, Kentucky in 2006, more than a quarter-century after the rule was adopted, featured a copilot so focused on a non-stop soliloquy of personal discussion that he hardly had time to run the checklists.[25] Then, too, there was a captain in that Comair cockpit with the responsibility to stop the chatter, but he made no attempt to do so. What I'm getting at, Will, is that when you butt heads with a professional, cultural bias as strong as the airline pilots' feeling about the freedom to say anything they wanted in their cockpits, it takes decades to change it and kill that bias, even when it's a federal regulation. For us in the OR? Same thing. Same impetus and inertia against change. We've now begun the same battle to quiet down the OR, and yet, fortunately, we don't have an FAA imposing such a rule and inflaming myopic resistance."

"So what *did* you do here?"

"We used our same consensus technique. We got the majority of our physicians out on a retreat, laid out the case for what we dubbed a chatter-free zone around the sterile field, and we wrangled and fought and spit and snarled among ourselves until the logical case became so overwhelming that they all grudgingly agreed to tone it down and approve the idea of videotaping every procedure."

"So, do they really comply with the no-conversation zone?"

"It's not a no-conversation zone, but it's a concept that we should only be discussing professional matters pertaining to the procedure before us. If the attending decides to say, 'Hey, Judy, how's your kid doing at Harvard?' no one's going to sound the alarm and call a deviation and jump on him. But this is where the videos become so useful, because an attending who has let the conversation drift too far as an emerging normalization of deviance, will catch it himself or herself on the next reviewed video."

"They review each *procedure*?"

"Oh, my, no! No one has that much time. But what we do require is that our attendings and every member of an OR team review the full video of one operation per month, and we even send a password-protected DVD disk home with them after they tell us which procedure they want to watch. If they see themselves chattering too much, they pull themselves back into line, for the most part. There are, of course, occasional exceptions that Alice has to deal with."

"Then, why didn't the same thing work with the pilots

regarding the sterile cockpit rules? Why didn't they police themselves?"

"Two reasons. First, no one was reviewing the audio tapes unless something went very wrong and the FAA and the company got involved. Second, in the case of pilots, the rules were imposed on them by an outside authority for which they had scant respect. In fact, even after the sterile cockpit practice and rule were accepted, it took almost 25 years for the pilots to realize how unsafe extraneous chatter in the cockpit can be. We did it the other way, inside out."

"So, same principle. If it's invented here and we've all agreed to it..."

"That's right. Then it can be enforced by peer pressure and personal commitment alone. Culture change is exponentially faster when the culture itself decides to make the change. Culture change by mandate from outside is always much slower and more problematic, with resistance a guaranteed byproduct."

"Understood."

"What I also hope you were witnessing today in that OR, Will, was a team taking the process far more seriously than they used to."

"It was strange, Jack, but you're right. There was a level of focus and trust there I've never really experienced. It was almost otherworldly. And the debrief was unprecedented as well. I thought for sure it would be hurried. This was the third case today for Jim Lyon, the attending. But after closing and finishing the paperwork, he waited until the team had finished their duties and sat down with some coffee and ran back through the procedure asking for any observations or proposed corrections, as well as whether they'd skipped something or changed any of the protocols. He went through the video, and that still blows me away that you tape the procedures and they're really reviewed. They stopped to zoom in so he could discuss the way they'd positioned a retractor. He even used a post-brief checklist that I guess he'd written himself. All that and he used up no more than an extra eight minutes, if that."

"Jim is working on a new checklist model for us. By the way, that's high-definition TV going directly to a large-capacity computer hard drive, not tape."

"Okay, well, the upshot is that they not only knew they'd done a good, solid job, they squeezed a few procedural ideas out of the post-brief, and just like my experience in the ER, tentatively changed their procedure on the spot. And, I have no doubt that if something had gone wrong in there, they would have handled it with the same calm precision. In fact, I was impressed that one of the pre-op procedures was to check the availability and communication lines to the airway code team."

"They explain our handoff policy as well?"

"Yes! The concept of never having a patient without an identified advocate or patient manager. That's an exceptionally good idea."

"Where it works best is when several docs are taking care of one patient. Our procedure keeps them from becoming lackadaisical about who is really on first, or whose name is listed as attending versus who's really responsible for the patient's overall care and wellbeing. If you're listed as attending, you absolutely must be the coordinator and guardian in deed and attention as well as in name. We call it the physician-manager system. What happens, as I'm sure you understand, is that specialists often don't feel qualified to take on the overall responsibility for a patient's welfare, yet too often they get listed as the attending without realizing they have the baton. But they're more comfortable and responsive when the physician accepting responsibility as the real attending coordinates the care. So we've installed a systemic approach that never lets a patient be without the immediate concerned oversight of one managing physician, regardless of how many specialists that one doc is juggling with respect to consults. And we train our docs to understand that the more consults they go shopping for, the greater the need to document everything and disseminate all the resulting information and thinking to every doc involved. Otherwise, good people lose track of patients. Always remember that the acuity levels today are vastly higher than they were just a decade back. In acute cases going sour fast, confusion over who has the baton, and who's planning what, can cost a life."

"It certainly can," Will said, wincing. "One of our patients, back when I was CEO, got so disgusted trying to get someone to take direct responsibility for his case and pain management, he called 9-1-1 and had himself taken by ambulance to another hospital, with the local media milking it for all it was worth. The embarrassment for us was visceral and my board was livid. But in truth, when they got him at the other institution, they had to rush him to surgery for a bowel obstruction we had missed entirely."

"He saved his own life then?"

"Yes, although we had good, concerned docs working on the case. But they were completely disorganized and making unwarranted and untested assumptions all over the place about who was talking to whom, who was thinking surgery or an additional MRI, and what drug therapy to try next. We did an extensive systemic review and came up with a host of better ways, but not quite as good as your system."

The waitress appeared with their steaks and they both set about attacking them in silence for a few minutes before Jack resumed the exchange.

"By the way, Will, we compensate our docs additionally for taking the point on a case as the patient manager. We also compensate them honestly and directly for on-call duties, which gives a solid incentive to be instantly available and appreciative of the arrangement."

"You mean, versus just assigning the on-call status to someone as an uncompensated duty just because they have privileges?"

Jack glanced at him. "So, did your hospital try to do it that way, too?"

"Yes. Big mistake," Will said, wincing at the memory. "I stepped in and changed it right after I took over, but the ruffled feathers among the various physician groups were everywhere, and we even lost a patient because one of the surgeons waited until the very last minute to show up. I'm still angry about it. A young Navy Seabee from a car wreck, with a wife and two kids, was bleeding to death internally with a young ER doc begging this vascular surgeon in no fewer than eight phone calls to please come in immediately. Three hours of total heroics by the ER physician, but he didn't have the expertise. The young man expired five minutes before that jerk waltzed in the door swinging his cell phone casually by the antenna, but I guess he made his point."

"What'd you do?"

"I overreacted and got rid of him on the spot, alienating the largest surgical group, and had to bring in two vascular surgeons at considerable expense to replace him. But when I calmed down and looked into the system, I was shocked that I'd never realized just how abusive we'd become to our physicians when we required them to be on call. We'd created and exacerbated our own problem."

"Will, there are some aspects of what we've done here in terms of change and focus that I want to make sure you're aware of. First, are you familiar with the statement that every system is perfectly designed to get the results it consistently achieves?"

"Yes."

"I think the import of that phrase is brilliant and vital. If a human system is routinely producing results you don't like, it's because that system is *perfectly designed* to give you just those results. So, if we're killing an average of 10 patients a year at Our Lady of Reasonably Good Outcomes Hospital, that's because that hospital's systems are *perfectly designed* to relieve 10 patients per year of their lives unnecessarily. If you want a different result, you have to redesign the system. That's the bedrock-basic of the patient safety crisis. Bad systems, not bad individuals, will give us unacceptable results consistently until we re-engineer that system. But the principle is the same for less-than-desirable levels of service quality, too. If you're not producing the quality you want — the quality you need in order to be a shining example of the best possible medical center — the culprit is your system, not your people."

"Bad or incompetent people can be a part of that systemic problem, though," Will added.

"Of course! But the traditional response, especially with a cultural bias toward finding one person to blame for anything that goes wrong, is to focus on bad components in the human organization, not bad design. That is always, categorically, a mistake. Don't like your service quality or your safety performance? Your problem is your entire system, not just your people."

"Understood. We need more wine?"

"Half a bottle of a good red is my limit. No, thanks. But back on the subject — the other stuff I wanted to mention goes to the heart of the first tier of defense against medical error impacting patients. Remember I said the first tier is to work to minimize human errors? Doing your best systemically to reduce the incidence of human mistake?"

"Yes. One of three."

"Right. Tier two is to build your system to *anticipate* the errors that will still occur and build enough buffers into the system to catch and cancel the effect of those errors in time. One method of doing that is creating a fully communicating and mutually supportive team focused on the common goal, a team that can catch together individual mistakes they can't prevent individually. Another method of tier two prophylaxis is bar-coding at the bedside. Both approaches fully expect errors. And, of course, the third tier is, after you've minimized error production and built in the buffers, you still assign only a maximum 50 percent expectation that everything is going to go as planned, so you're ready and sensitive to any indication of failure."

"I think I have it memorized now, Jack."

"I'm sure you do. But here's the deal, back to tier one: Human errors, as inevitable as they are, don't happen in a vacuum. We can increase or decrease the probability of human error by the way we take care of ourselves. It doesn't mean if we're well-rested and well-fed we can then be perfect, but it does mean that there are factors we can personally control about ourselves that will further reduce the possibility of making a major mistake."

"I need a clearer picture, Jack. You're talking about being more careful by being more healthy?"

"No, not really. I'm talking about not coming to work in a condition that increases your potential for errors. We can help our people lessen the possibility of making significant mistakes by training them to use better procedures and to have a greater understanding of how errors are made, but if that physician or nurse, or whoever, is at the same time unaware of the performance problems that hunger, dehydration, fatigue, emotional distraction, and even things like 'multi-tasking' can create, then we're accepting — wiring in — a historical engine of error production."

"So, you train those basics?"

"Oh, better than that. We use part of a new approach system called the Global War on Error, a program developed for the U.S. Marines and their aviators and used very successfully in corporate aviation as well.[26] What that instructional approach does is focus the individual professional on the reality that as carbon-based humans, we have very real physical limitations that directly affect our performance. Just like pilots are taught not to exceed the limitations of their air machines, we have a responsibility not to exceed the limitations of our carbon-based bodies, especially if we're expecting ourselves to perform at optimum levels."

"And this is a new approach?"

"Hey, as a resident, you were indefatigable, right?"

"Well, I was supposed to be."

"Thirty hours on duty, no problem. That's how we're all told we should be."

"Agreed. And at that point, you're young enough to handle it."

"Ah, Will, but that's the thing, you see. You're not. That was a bill of goods they sold us, a fraudulent expectation. What's that phrase from the movie *Top Gun*? They encouraged us to write checks our bodies couldn't cash? You and I never were invulnerable to fatigue. When we were dead tired, we were performing at a far lower level of efficiency and intellect, and after a certain point, we were just plain dangerous as young docs. Do you realize we now have hard research that if a person is kept awake more than 21 hours, his or her performance is below that of someone with a blood alcohol level of .08?"[27]

"Legally drunk?"

"Yes! Legally schnockered! You want your kid or significant other operated on by a drunken doc? Of course not, yet the number of times an extremely fatigued surgeon has picked up a scalpel and started work on a patient — a physician with the equivalent of .08 alcohol in his bloodstream — probably can be measured in the millions. It's the way we always did things!"

"So, you've instituted an aggressive program against staff fatigue?"

"There again, we had to get our docs and nurses deep into the data to convince them that we had to change. But, you see, that's just a starting point. Dehydration, as simple as that seems, can also produce anomalous behavior, as can poor nutrition, and I'm talking about serious degradation in performance over just a few days of abuse. The figures they use based on hard research about all these physical elements are really startling. I never knew how little it took to become dehydrated, let alone cumulatively fatigued."

"You mentioned multi-tasking, too."

"Absolutely. We can't physically do it."

"Now, Jack, I happen to be pretty good at multi-tasking."

"No, you just think you are. What you're really good at is *sequential*-tasking, because humans, unlike digital computers, cannot run conscious mental programs in parallel — only in sequence. We just get very good at darting our attention from one thing to another and back again in such a way that it feels like we're parallel processing."

"Don't pilots multi-task in instrument flying?"

"I always thought they did, and thousands of them think they do to this day. But in reality, when they're reading instruments in fog, for instance, their concentration is sequential. This instrument, then that instrument, then back again. The reason for making this such a point, Will, is that sequential-taskers versus multi-taskers have a grave vulnerability. If you overload them — if they try to handle too many things at once, bouncing back and forth among those tasks, like reading instruments or a nurse trying to juggle six or more patients — they can reach task saturation. And when you task-saturate someone, instead of just slowing him down, all the balls that person is juggling fall to the mental floor at once. The whole picture crashes, and like a computer freezing up and resetting, you've got to start everything up again. This is why air traffic controllers have to limit the number of aircraft they're working with and talking to, and it's a lesson we've just not inculcated into our culture. We task-saturate nurses every day in American health care, and then fire them when they turn human on us and forget something critical. We task-saturate doctors, especially if they're fatigued or distracted, and then we think they're less than good practitioners because they couldn't tough it out and perform flawlessly."

"This is fascinating and not a little disturbing."

"I tell you, Will, when you've sat through a course on personal error prevention, especially the parts about our human limitations, you come away shaken by how many times in the past your own inabilities have been not the result of laziness or mental limitations, but just pure physical limits. They also teach a great course about error-producing attitudes, such as the attitude that the rules are for average people and I'm above average so I don't need the rules.[28] But with just the part on physiological and psychological maintenance, the truth is we push ourselves too far and for all our touted knowledge of the human body we docs in particular act as if we were androids, not humans. We act like we're invulnerable to such physical limitations as fatigue and hunger and dehydration and emotional upsets. What's the culture code for doctors? Hero.[29] Can heroes get fatigued? Heck, no. Superman doesn't fall victim to fatigue, and we've been wearing the equivalent of a mental red 'S' all our careers."

"What's the culture code for nurses?"

"Mother. Martyr. Saint. Selfless. Which is why what you're going to experience tomorrow morning in being on the floor, and working alongside our nurses, is so important. We've had to reengineer the culture codes for doctors and nurses and get them to speak the same language, and that's been perhaps the toughest thing we've faced. In fact, the education experiences of nurses and doctors are so profoundly different that neither knows what the other really does. Doctors get upset at nurses all the time for not understanding what they, the docs, do. But they don't realize how little they know of what their nurses have been taught to do and understand. In addition, a nurse today is vastly more sophisticated than a nurse 50 years ago. Today our nurses are carrying stethoscopes, sometimes far more than our physicians. But let me save all that for your morning session."

Jack was looking around for the waitress and finally caught her eye.

"You game for some coffee?"

"Absolutely. By the way, who's shepherding me around in the morning?"

"One of our nurse managers, Patti Miller. She's incredible, but you knew I was going to say that."

Will grinned. "I suspected."

"Here's the thing to keep in mind. Nurses are the point of contact that make all the difference in quality of care, patient and family impressions and the overall welfare of our patient. The work of the most brilliant surgeon on the planet can be destroyed by an inattentive nurse in a bad system, and the system we used to have absolutely hard-wired major systemic errors into each and every aspect of the world our nurses inhabited. We've changed that world, we've changed the rules, we've swallowed big cost increases in providing the right number of nurses and the right people for the job, we've changed the way the job assignments and patient assignments are done, and a hundred other things I think you'll find unique."

"I see they're wearing uniforms, too."

"That was their choice, with our encouragement, but it's raised the professional pride levels — especially the modern uniform they helped design. Also, I should tell you, one of the missions we, as a hospital, have committed to is ending the mass confusion over what it takes to educate a professional nurse. Two-year degree, three-, or four-, gets you the same RN status and the same job across the nation. That's absurd and that has to end, and we're hammering away at it. But I'll let Patti tell you about it."

"Okay."

"Right now I want to ask you a personal question."

"Sure, Jack."

"What the heck happened at that hospital you ran? I see a smart, dedicated, empathetic man of medicine across the table who's taken his own time to learn all about how to change the medical world, and I've heard a few references you've made to something that happened. Will you tell me?"

Will knew the look of strain had crossed his face, erasing the smile that had been there moments before. It was always painful reliving it, regardless of how clinical his analysis, but he'd expected the question and already decided that Jack deserved a full answer. The waitress was sliding the check carefully onto the middle of the table and Will snatched it a little too aggressively.

"Hey, Will, let me take that."

"No way. After all the training you've provided and the hospitality?"

"No pun intended."

Will looked puzzled, but finally caught the pun. "Oh! Right. Hospitality. But, no, this one's mine."

"Well, thank you. Great meal." Jack watched Will slip his credit card into the check folder and hand it to the waitress before looking back at St. Michael's CEO, who fixed him with an unwavering gaze. "You were just starting to tell me what happened."

"Right. Well, in a nutshell," Will began, "the hospital I ran killed my best friend's son, and I guess I'm on an eternal quest to figure out everything we did wrong, and everything we should have done that we didn't know how to do."

Jack was nodding but saying nothing, and Will continued.

"Ronnie Nolan was 11 and already one heck of kid. Talented baseball player, straight-A student and a bundle of energy. Wayne, his dad, and I had grown up best friends, chased women together, gone to college together, and even before Ronnie was conceived, Wayne and Cindy, his wife, asked me to be a godparent. Anyway, suffice it to say that Wayne, who was, still is, an airline captain, looked to me for medical advice. So when little Ronnie ended up hurting himself in an after-school fight and wrestling match, Wayne called me and I had him bring Ronnie to our ER. When he came in, he was in severe pain, and Wayne told me he thought his shoulder was broken and displaced. I couldn't verify it on examination and our emergency resident couldn't either. We had an X-ray, of course, and it just didn't show a break, and frankly, I had some experience with Wayne trying to play doctor before, so I explained to him that the evidence wasn't there.

"Our docs sent him home with his dad and a lot of pain medication, but things didn't seem to get much better. I had Wayne bring him back in for an MRI as soon as I heard Ronnie was complaining of numbness in his right arm, and I arranged a quick referral to the best vascular surgeon we had. At my personal request our vascular doc took a hard look and reported back that he didn't see anything serious, and since by that time the pain and the numbness had subsided, he postulated that maybe a little sports rehab would solve the problem. So now we had X-rays and an MRI and no indication of any physical problem, although Wayne kept telling me he was sure Ronnie's scapula was a bit lower on the right side. You know us, if it doesn't show in the X-ray, then it doesn't exist, and that's what we all hung our hats on. That and the fact that a non-physician was trying to convince us of something we had already discounted. But one evening months later Wayne calls terribly concerned and says Ronnie's right arm is blue, numb and cold. I have him rush to our ER and I met them there. One of our techs does a Doppler, but we don't discover until later that this guy is not competent and he failed to go high enough, and therefore found nothing. Ronnie's case is handed off to the incoming resident who fails to read the notes, doesn't discuss it with the outbound resident or the nurse, and comes in to tell us that there's no indication of circulatory problems. Maybe, he says, Ronnie just slept on it wrong. Wayne blows up and I'm not far behind. I jump in the middle of it, alienating the resident, order a new X-ray, Doppler and MRI all at once, and hours later we finally get the vascular guy to come in. Much to everyone's shock, we discover that there was a break in the clavicle months before and we completely missed it.

"Wayne, in other words, had been right from the start, and even with me looking out for Ronnie and commandeering my own hospital, I couldn't get us to look far enough. In fact, we missed more than the break. The broken clavicle had displaced and had been pressing down on the subclavian vein and brachial plexus supply for months, and Ronnie, as a result, had developed a potentially lethal clot a half-inch away from his heart. We admit him immediately and the vascular surgeon schedules the OR for 7 a.m. and goes home to get some sleep. The decision to delay until morning is a mistake we didn't catch, since he should have gone to surgery immediately and another vascular surgeon should have been paged in. Our attending's plan is to surgically remove the clot with the appropriate safeguards, and then see about rebreaking, lifting and wiring, if necessary, the clavicle. But in the admitting process and in the handoff to the floor, a vital cautionary warning doesn't get posted properly. The warning that under no circumstances should a blood pressure cuff be used on Ronnie's right arm does not get posted at bedside when he arrives on the floor. The warning is clearly the very first order in the chart, because to do so would dislodge the clot and potentially kill him. He's taken to the floor, but before his dad and I can even get up there, a traveling nurse covering what to her is an unfamiliar med/surg floor, gets him comfortable. But then, without referring to our new policy which demands inspection of the chart before anything is done on vitals, she puts on a cuff to take the blood pressure and pumps it up. To her it's as much of a ritual as breathing. But the cuff pressure immediately dislodges the entire clot, which shoots into his heart like a runaway freight train, fragmenting as it goes, shards blocking various arteries while a large piece heads for his brain and essentially shuts down the blood supply. In short, within seconds he's crashing, and his brain is dying. We walk in just as she's calling the code with no clue what happened. All of us tried desperately to get him back for over 40 minutes, and it's not until much later that we discover that he's brain dead. In other words, we lost him."

"Yikes."

"I simply can't erase the horror of that moment. It plays over and over in my head like a skipping CD, my lifelong buddy standing there in tears saying, 'Do something! C'mon, DO something!' But there's nothing else I can think to do. We're standing there looking like deer in the headlights, and to his father it looks like a willingness to just stop trying, like we might be too tired."

"You did a lengthy root cause analysis, right?"

"Oh, yeah. And that's what nearly killed me. So many mistakes, so many lost opportunities on handoffs, so little reality between what I thought our people were doing to comply with the directed patient safety changes and procedures and what they were really doing. I thought my institution was so much safer than it was. The traveler, for instance, had simply done things the way she'd always done them at other institutions. No one had bothered to tell her she couldn't practice in our hospital without sitting at the nurses' station for five minutes and reading the basic rules for travelers. Why? It was someone else's responsibility, and the charge nurse wasn't about to take on someone else's work."

"And," Jack added, "the staff, not being the drivers of those changes, didn't think about making it everyone's responsibility to instruct a floater or traveler, right?"

"Right. I see that now. Clearly."

Both men fell silent for a few very long seconds, the scene almost replaying on the wall before them before Jack sighed and spoke.

"Will, there's a limit to kicking yourself for a systems failure, even in this terrible circumstance."

"You're missing something, though, Jack. See, I was part of the problem personally. The CEO steps in and gets in the way of everyone trying to get my godson better care. I later found at least five points at which my interference caused more problems than it solved. I can't say Ronnie wouldn't have died if I had stayed out of it, but maybe he wouldn't have been rushed to the floor and mishandled if I hadn't been cracking a whip. So, my hospital, my watch, my docs, my own expertise as a physician, and we screwed it up over and over until we killed him. If he'd been at St. Michael's, he would have lived, even if you'd missed the broken clavicle."

"Okay, Will," Jack said, downing the last of his coffee and standing slowly. Will pocketed the receipt and stood as well.

"Human systems, Will, are always works in progress. As tough a reality as it is, your godson's crash was just like most of the airline crashes of the past 20 years — shocking and terrible occurrences that nevertheless spawn important changes that end up saving many more lives in the future. Not one of those deaths in Tenerife was in vain, for instance, because thousands have been saved by the revolution in aviation safety that would not have happened otherwise. The process of flying an airplane or a hospital is messy, but ultimately worth everything, provided we learn the lessons only once."

Will's Notes:

The concept of videotaping every procedure and leaving control of the tapes in the hands of the physicians can be a powerful tool for self-correction, especially self-correction of demeanor, behavior, and just the way one comes across to your team-mates. Jack made the point that airline pilots have been using this technique with great success for years, and that if you're not a professional communicator, you have no real idea of how you come across, especially under pressure.

Using a post-brief after each surgery, especially with a short checklist, enables a surgical team to capture even subtle and easily-forgotten lessons learned.

The Physician Manager System used by St. Michael's guaran-tees someone is always in charge of, and on top of, a particular patient's care. The important thing is, the manager is not just in titular charge of the patient's care, this is a real, hands-on, around the clock level of responsibility, with full expectation that the nurses will call the physician manager at any time if there is any question or suspected problem. The patient also has full and immediate access to the manager.

The quote often used by Dr. Don Berwick: "Every system is perfectly designed to get the results it consistently achieves." i.e., if a hospital is killing 10 patients per year, it is perfectly designed to do just that. To reduce the carnage, the system has to be profoundly changed.

The three tiers of a Safety System are:

1. Minimize the occurrence of human error through training, system changes, and education as well as cultural change;

2. Despite #1, expect human mistakes and build your system to fully absorb every anticipatable mistake without patient impact (much the same as aircraft manufacturers build in backup systems to backup the backup system);

3. Even with #1 and #2 complete, the third step is to thor-oughly redirect the thinking of all team members so as to

assign a 50/50 chance of serious error at any given time in a patient's care (given that the normal expectation after Tiers 1 and 2 is to expect a 90 % probability of error-free performance).

- Despite our constant citation of multi-tasking as an admirable human trait, humans cannot multi-task. Instead, we sequentially task, which means that if we task-saturate ourselves to the point of dysfunction, all current tasks a person is trying to do at once are disrupted.

- Culture code for physicians: Hero. Culture code for Nurses: Mother, martyr and saint.

CHAPTER THIRTEEN

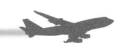

Enough for tonight — I'm emotionally exhausted!

Will looked at his last entry in the already overfilled legal pad. He'd tried to concentrate and write down some of the things Jack had advocated at dinner about personal error producing factors, but reliving the loss of Ronnie Nolan was too great a distraction. Jack had listened compassionately and then, realizing how fresh the wounds were, tried to redirect the conversation to patient safety matters as he drove Will back to the hotel.

It hadn't worked.

Eight fifty-five p.m., Will noted, looking at his watch. He should force himself to keep working. Instead, he found himself flipping on the TV and leaving it to blare while he took a hot shower, as if the hot water could wash away the self-recrimination that always flowed so easily from the memories. Properly numbed, at least physically, he dried off, doused the lights, and shut down the TV after setting the alarm for 6 a.m.

But sleep was impossible. A half-hour of tossing around convinced him, and he snapped the lights on again and dressed, digging through the bottom of his bag for the tube carrying a high-quality cigar he'd been hoarding. Cigarettes had never been a temptation, but cigars were, and he allowed himself a few every month, especially on clear, warm nights with no wind and a sky full of stars overhead. Reflective time, he'd dubbed it, as if a prescription was needed to justify the indulgence.

The network show Jack had mentioned — *Boston Legal* — had been kindling a hunger for more of those evenings with a varietal cigar and a single-malt scotch, much the same as the two main characters used at the end of each episode.

Will opened the mini-bar, pleased to find at least a low-grade single-malt in the form of two miniatures which he emptied into a pedestrian water glass. He pulled on a jacket and took the newly-snipped cigar outside on the hotel lawn to a large chair. With the rich smoke curling comfortably into the clear sky and the warmth of the scotch, he forced all the other thoughts and regrets from his mind and began replaying some of the stories Jack had told.

It seemed for every terrible tale of accidental medical injury or death he'd experienced personally, Jack knew of two or three more that were even more upsetting. The loss of the young Navy man at the hands of an angry vascular surgeon at Will's hospital always kindled a flash of anger, but Jack's story of a California disaster had been even more disturbing.

"An old friend called in a marker during a medical symposium in L.A.," Jack had begun, "and I let myself get roped into counseling the very shaken staff of the day surgery center he owned. So I stayed over for an evening and went out to this beautiful facility, and they had a nice dinner catered and I spoke to the nurses and the woman who served as director. A tragic mistake well over a year before had killed a patient and they just weren't recovering. Half the nurses had left, but the half that remained — those who had been there when the death occurred — were still in post-traumatic stress. An otherwise healthy 18-year-old had arrested on the table when the anesthesiologist reached for Decadrone but mistakenly drew up and injected 10cc's of Epinephrine. They had never had a code at that surgery center and both the staff and the docs were totally unprepared.

"By the time they finally began to get organized, the patient was gone. A huge lawsuit ensued, and everyone testified in lockstep that it was a tragic human mistake that led to a mix-up in the vials. The plaintiffs settled, since nothing outrageous had happened, and everyone had apparently done their best to save the boy. Well, I spent two hours with these folks ostensibly to discuss patient safety methods, but in reality I spent the time trying to get them to forgive themselves. I'm heading out the door when one of the nurses comes up to me and says in an almost inaudible voice, 'They lied.' She motions me outside and tells me the nurses who were in the OR with her that day lied in their depositions when they supported the anesthesiologist's version of what happened. Yes, he had grabbed the wrong vial as he filled the hypodermic, but instead of the image he and the attending had painted of super-serious medicine men concentrating hard on the patient's welfare, as the anesthesiologist was drawing up the wrong medication and injecting it, he was also balancing his cell phone on his shoulder and talking to his stockbroker to order a stock sale. The judge, the jury, the lawyers, and my friend, the owner of the center, had never known the truth. And the nurses who lied about it? She told me they did so because the anesthesiologists' multi-specialty medical group accounted for more than 75 percent of the surgery center's business, and they were convinced telling the truth would have meant the loss of all their jobs."

Will shook his head and sipped some more scotch, wondering how either of those two physicians could ever pass a mirror again without turning away. Jack, he could tell, was still torn over the revelation, and very unsure whether he'd done the right thing by honoring the nurse's impassioned request to say nothing.

Winking position lights on a passing business jet broke his concentration, a flight out of nearby Broomfield, he figured, headed east. The sight of the jet brought back the other story Jack had taken him through in minute detail, a galvanizing occurrence Will vaguely recalled but now wanted to know more about. It was, Jack had said, perhaps the most effective teaching accident in recent commercial airline history.

The moonless night of February 12, 1989, had set the stage when approximately 60 miles south of Honolulu, Hawaii, the large cargo door on the right forward fuselage of a United Airlines Boeing 747 suddenly blew out into the night.

"The flight was at 23,000 feet," Jack had said, explaining the fact that it was low enough for everyone aboard to stay conscious for a few minutes without oxygen. "Had they been way up at cruise altitude, we would have lost them all, because the oxygen system failed.

"Before departure in Honolulu, the cargo door latching mechanism had suffered a mechanical failure and was not completely locked. As the pressure increased inside the climbing Boeing, the latching mechanism failed suddenly, the considerable pressure inside the aircraft propelling the door outward as it ripped a large portion of the aircraft fuselage above the hinge and ripped nine seats out of the coach cabin with passengers still strapped in them.

"Suddenly a four-engine jumbo jet that had departed weighing over 750,000 pounds was down to two operating engines on the left wing, and they were trying to fly a tangle of structural damage on the right side. The airplane was completely depressurized, and the 'explosion' had also ripped out both the passenger and crew oxygen systems along with the intercom wiring. The pilots way up on the flight deck on the second floor of the 747 had no way of talking to the flight attendants on the shattered main deck, which was now open to the darkness and the rushing airstream outside. Several of the passengers who had been lucky enough *not* to be yanked to their deaths through the hole, sat now with their feet dangling over the abyss as the crew, unsure what had happened, turned the big airplane back toward Honolulu and tried in vain to get oxygen to their masks as they started an emergency descent. The copilot declared an emergency as the captain — who was two months away from retirement — fought the bucking aircraft down to a more oxygen-rich altitude. But the captain's attempt to level the aircraft at 10,000 feet wasn't working. A 747 can fly level at heavy weight even on one engine. But the aerodynamic damage on the right side of United Flight 811 was so great (and the additional drag so elevated), they could not stay level without running out of flying speed. With the captain pushing the nose over and the big jet descending at nearly 1,200 feet per minute at 280 knots some 50 miles from Honolulu International Airport, the situation was grim at best.

"Even without running the math the crew understood that if the descent rate remained anywhere close to the same, they would hit the dark waters of the Pacific Ocean in 8 minutes still some 15 miles south of the island of Oahu. The captain, mean-while, was task-saturated and focusing all his cognitive skill on trying to hang onto the bucking jumbo jet. Had their safety depended, as it once did, on the captain barking out orders and directing the recovery effort as if John Wayne were at the controls, the recovery attempt would have failed immediately. The captain had nothing left to use on planning and reasoning, so great was the basic challenge of just keeping the 747 in the air."

Will took another drink of scotch and realized he'd almost drained the glass. Jack's point had been crystal clear, and it was already an accident Will wanted to memorize. Something *had* obviously changed with dramatic import at United between the late '70s and that night in 1989, and he thought about Jack's impassioned narrative.

"I tell you, Will," he'd said, his hands in the air over the dinner table demonstrating what he'd been told it would take to hang onto a crippled 747, "if that copilot and flight engineer hadn't had the new crew resource management training and the discipline and culture change thoroughly welded into their thinking, and their reactions, they would have sat there like so many others over time waiting in vain for an overloaded captain to give them clear direction. That wouldn't have happened, so the only way the subordinates were going to speak up was after the cultural overhaul."

"So the copilot spoke up?" Will had prompted.

"Both the copilot and the flight engineer were in lockstep, helping the captain without being asked. That wouldn't have happened 10 years before. But United's captains were now required to be leaders, not just commanders, and required to fully incorporate the intellect of their subordinate crewmembers, who had been equally trained to speak up without hesitation when something needed to be said. In addition, the second officer — traditionally the silent member of the crew — had been told that he was equally responsible for the lives of everyone aboard, and that if something had to be done for safety, he was to challenge the pilots twice, and then do it himself if they didn't respond. So, the copilot was firing off heading information to keep the captain on course back for Honolulu, and they were all scared out of their minds! I mean, I wouldn't want to fly with pilots in that kind of situation if they weren't scared to some extent.

"Despite the fact that all three of these guys were veterans of flying United jets around Hawaii, at one point one of the pilots turns around and says, 'See if there are any other airports between here and Honolulu!' Of course, unless there happened to be a very large aircraft carrier between them and Honolulu there was nothing out there but water, and the big jet was descending steadily toward it, pulled down by the weight, which included the weight of the large fuel load they were carrying. Now, the second officer — the flight engineer — realized this, and he tried three times to impart that critical piece of information to his task-saturated captain in order to get permission to begin dumping fuel. 'Lots of fuel, should we dump?' he asks the copilot, but neither the captain nor the copilot really hear him, they're so utterly distracted and overloaded. Finally, after what must have seemed an eternity to the engineer, the copilot realizes what the engineer has been trying to say, turns around and says, 'Start dumping the fuel.' 'I AM dumping,' the engineer says, because in accordance with CRM training he's challenged the situation more than twice and then proceeded to make it happen in order to keep them in the air. And what he did was the first of two times the second officer saves the airplane that night. Now, with the fuel dump system spewing 5,000 pounds a minute into the night, they're getting lighter with every precious second. Ten years before, the act of turning on those pumps without a direct order from the captain would have been very risky for the engineer's career. But by changing the culture and empowering the engineer, United had given this crew a fighting chance of working as a team and finding a way to stay aloft long enough to get back to the airport."

"They were still descending?" Will had asked.

"Yes, although more slowly," Jack had replied. "Now, as they descended through 7,000 feet above the water, the engineer asks if he should run downstairs and check the situation, since they can't talk to the flight attendants. This time the captain says yes, and the engineer gets up and leaves the flight deck, descends the circular staircase to the main deck, and returns, all in less than 45 seconds. Out of breath and profoundly shaken, he tells the captain, 'The right side is gone from about the, ah, one-right, back! It's just open! You're just lookin' outside!' 'Waddaya mean, pieces?' the captain asks. 'Looks like a bomb. The fuselage, it's just open!' The captain asks, 'Is anyone...' and he can't finish the sentence, but the second officer understands completely. 'I don't know...' replies the shaken engineer, 'some people are probably gone... I can't tell...' Now, the 747 is still coming down, pilots call it drifting down, and at around 6,000 feet the copilot turns to the captain and says, 'What a thing to happen on your second to... ah... last month.' And the captain, still holding a death grip on the yoke and fighting to keep the wings level, says 'No s– – –!'"

Will and Jack had both laughed at the incongruous comic relief in a moment of near blind panic in the air.

"With 24 miles to go," Jack continued, "they reached a decision point. Pilots of large airplanes have always been taught that if they ever have to ditch — put their airplane down in the water — they'd better do it in a controlled way with a plan; otherwise they will surely kill themselves and everyone aboard. This crew hasn't yet accepted the fact that they may have to ditch. They haven't done a single checklist exactly right, and at 4,000 feet, remembering that they were sinking at over 1,000 feet per minute what seemed a few miles back, the captain loses faith that they have a chance of making land. 'I don't know if we're gonna make this,' he says. 'Ah... I can't... hold altitude.' Now, up until this point the copilot has been very positive, helping the captain along with headings and information and talking to the controller in Honolulu, but suddenly he sees the hideous probability, too, that they may have to fly into the Pacific Ocean with a crippled jumbo jet that Boeing later said would have ripped apart on impact. Suddenly the copilot is so shaken he can't get a sentence out of his mouth. 'Okay...' he stammers, '... ah... we're 24 miles out... and... ah... we're driftin' down slowly... so...' And this is the moment in the transcript of the cockpit voice recorder that's just staggering, Will," Jack had said, his eyes flashing, coming forward in his chair and gesturing across the table.

"Everything we teach our physicians about setting up an environment in which the most junior member is not just asked, but is required to speak up immediately if there's any hint of a problem, and everything we do to bring our formerly cowed nurses up to the point where they would never hesitate to say to even the most senior surgeon, 'Doctor, I think you may be about to cut the wrong thing,' and here's the shining proof of how effective such a cultural change can be. The captain is split-seconds away from a decision to prepare for ditching, and the first officer's resistance has crumbled, when the crewmember who used to be taught to shut up and never, ever challenge a captain, the second officer, even though he has a much better grasp on the dynamics of what's happening, leans forward and says, 'You're gonna make it!' just like that. The captain, on the transcript, says 'Huh?' And the second officer repeats it, 'You're gonna make it!' 'Well,' says the copilot, his mind obviously reeling from hope to despair and back, 'make sure we don't hit any @$!%# hills on the way in,' and the second officer all but cuts him off, saying 'There aren't any hills!' And as a direct result of the active interjection of the most junior crewmember, they decide to continue on and not try to ditch. Now, see, the second officer knew that their descent rate had been reduced to almost nothing, but the two guys up front were so overwhelmed they didn't see it. Together the three of them made the decisions that saved every life left aboard. By himself, the captain would have ditched, and most likely more than 300 people would have died on impact or drowned. One person, one voice, changed everything. And that was only possible because the airline had changed its culture."

"And they made it?" Will had asked.

"They had one shot at it and only one. If they'd tried to do a go-around with only two engines and all that damage, they would have ended up impacting upside down in the middle of Honolulu. But as they got closer to the airport and managed to get some flaps extended and the landing gear down, they realized they were high enough that they were, in fact, going to make it. The engineer had been right. Of course, there's another hilarious moment when they're about five miles out and everything's looking good. Remember, they've got a hole in the side of the fuselage as big as Tulsa where the cargo door blew away and ripped up the side of the airplane. The copilot, trying to make sure they haven't forgotten anything, turns to the second officer suddenly and asks, 'Are we depressurized?' Moments later they touch down safely and manage to stop, and all but the nine passengers blown outside lived to tell about it."[30]

The cigar was down to the last inch, Will realized, and the scotch was long-since drained. He pulled his mind back from the traumatized cockpit of United 811 to refocus on the stars overhead, feeling a sudden chill in the Colorado evening as he glanced at his watch, feeling tired at last.

Eleven thirty p.m.

Patti Miller would be waiting for him at 7 a.m.

CHAPTER FOURTEEN

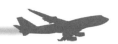

"You're no longer an active hospital CEO?" Patti Miller was reading Will's face closely as she stood in front of the charge nurse station on 4 West.

"Not anymore," he replied, feeling uncomfortable in the unflinching focus of her large eyes. She'd been waiting at the elevator for him, somehow alerted he was on his way up, and Will had recognized her immediately.

"A true force of nature," had been Jack's description. "Five-foot-seven, full head of cascading chestnut hair, a perpetual, sincere smile, two master's degrees and now working on her Ph.D. She also comes equipped with the most intense green eyes I've ever seen. She's a formidable intellect, Will, and she's been more than instrumental in redesigning nursing here at St. Michael's, and, we hope, creating a template for the rest of the medical world."

Will met Patti's eyes again, thinking Jack had understated his description of her intensity.

"So, Dr. Jenkins..."

"Will, please."

"Thank you, Will. And I'm Patti, and we're all first-names up here. But I'm curious. You're not a CEO currently, yet you're here for several days spending time with us and working hard to learn how we're different," she added a raised eyebrow.

"Well, let's just say that, when I was running a hospital, I was never able to achieve anything close to what you've created here, and when I heard about you, I wanted to learn."

Patti nodded knowingly. "I think you'll definitely be a CEO again, and a good one if you take enough notes."

"I will?" he chuckled.

"You won't be able to help yourself, once we've thoroughly assimilated you into this philosophy. And there are too many hospitals in desperate need of good people to change them." She waved at someone down the corridor and turned back to him. "Ready?"

"Absolutely."

"I wanted you to see our morning handoff. Others would call it report, but that doesn't accurately describe the way we approach it."

"You gather here at the charge nurse desk?"

"Yes, for an overall briefing. The LPNs... well, I'm getting a bit ahead of myself so let me just have you observe, and then we'll follow the individual nurses around as they hand off to their incoming counterparts."

Will followed her into a spacious central nurses station, noting the presence of five women and one man wearing comfortable white uniforms. She introduced Will to each of them by first name as other nurses arrived, each bearing up to five patient charts. While they arranged themselves around the interior of the station, he glanced at the array of flat computer screens, noting the presence of a familiar-looking physician computer order entry system and a single fax machine flanked by docking stations for an array of personal digital assistants, all of the same make and model.

Brenda, the incoming charge nurse for the day shift, went through a short briefing dealing with supply issues and read follow-up replies from various departments in the hospital on several problems reported by the staff over the previous 24 hours. The tone of the replies, Will realized, was not quite apologetic, but it was as if the various sectors of the hospital actually revolved around nursing, from transport to housekeeping, and were actually concerned about the nurses' opinions as each reported back through Brenda on some shortcoming. Each one included a quick systems analysis of how the problem had apparently occurred, what they were doing to make sure it didn't re-occur, and a request for after-action feedback from whichever nurse had brought the problem to their attention. It was all a bit bizarre, Will thought, but obviously not to the people around him, who were taking notes and making suggestions as if such supportive attitudes from the surrounding departments of a hospital were only natural.

He had expected at least a brief reference to every patient on the floor, but curiously, only the patients with emergent needs were mentioned, and then by first and last name, not room number.

Almost as quickly as they had convened, the group broke up, and Patti escorted Will down the corridor and into one of the private rooms.

At least, he had assumed it was a private room.

Instead, the door opened onto a suite of sorts containing five beds with sliding opaque glass walls dividing each bed from the next. Each bedroom was the equivalent of a private room in size. Three of the five had windows, but at the foot of each bed was an open curtain and, 10 feet distant, a semi-circular nurses station sat in full view, as if the entire array was a miniature ICU. The feel of each alcove, each roomette, was normal, except for the lack of four walls. Each had hanging, flat screen TVs, comfortable chairs for friends and family, and the usual array of instruments and spigots behind the bed.

Patti was smiling at Will's confused look. "I'll explain in a minute. For now just watch," she said in a low voice.

Two of the RNs who had attended the handoff briefing were now inside the small suite and conferring at the nurses desk — a small, high-tech console. They discussed several of the patients and their charts before the outgoing nurse handed over an electronic device the size of a large PDA. The two of them then began rounding on each of the five patients, the outbound nurse essentially doing a patient-by-patient handoff to her replacement before leaving, but involving each patient in the details of the handoff. Will could hear laughter and personal exchanges with the patients and family members throughout the process, and a goodbye wave at the door brought the same response from four of the five occupants.

Will and Patti followed the departing nurse into the hallway to talk.

"For some reason," Patti began with a knowing smile, "I figured you just might have a few questions."

"I'm not sure where to begin," he replied, shaking his head. "I wasn't expecting a small ICU. Is this the only one on the floor?"

"Well, it's not an ICU. And all our rooms are like that."

"So it's a ward, sort of?"

"Not really, except for the 20 single rooms we keep on the third floor for isolation. But for everyone else, when we admit them to our hospital, we admit them to a community, and the individual members of a community should not be isolated. It's amazing how much better people do when they're around others." She motioned him into a large, carpeted break room and drew two cups of coffee before sitting at what could pass for a small boardroom table.

"You mind if I anticipate some of your questions, Will?"

"Not at all. Please."

"Okay, first, did the hospital you ran handle nursing staff issues the traditional way, by dictating exactly how many nurses were to be on every floor day-by-day, and setting in concrete how many hours they could work?"

"Yes, and with all the budget pressures it was continuously problematic, Patti. I did my best to give our nurse-managers more flexibility by asking for their monthly input on how many nurses they should have on each unit, but, frankly, no matter what we gave them, they wanted more. I think it's endemic."

She let the statement pass and continued. "What standards did you require of your nurse-managers in terms of the level of quality and patient satisfaction you wanted to see produced by their units?"

"We set a high standard for safety, then quality. We pushed them as hard as we could to realize that the hospital's fortunes were their fortunes, and that if our patients and our community thought we weren't a quality outfit, the census would drop off and we'd need fewer nurses."

"So, produce the highest quality or else?"

"Well, not that harsh, but that was the reality we lived with. I believed in being very frank with everyone, and I was, at least about the fact that all it would take is one very publicly injured or killed patient, and we could conceivably lose the hospital."

She was nodding. "We, as an institution, were also handing down a finite number of hours and dictating how many nurses could be here and requiring grids, and yet the sad truth is that we were ignorant of a very finite reality that I'm sure your hospital shared. We simply couldn't produce the level of service, safety, and patient satisfaction we needed with the resources we were allowing our people. It was impossible, and we had never opened our ears from the top to hear that reality from the front lines. Worse, our nurses never felt in charge or empowered, so they just hunkered down and plodded on, especially when repeated requests for relief to the 'C' suite were essentially ignored. Patient care, quality of care, and human attitudes had always been dictated from the top down, but it had never worked."

"So, we've shared the same basic experience. But how..."

She was holding a finger up to stop him. "The system we were using was as nonsensical as an airline knowing a particular flight requires at least 100,000 pounds of jet fuel, yet ordering the captain to go with only 60,000 because gas is so expensive. The alarmed captain tells you it won't work, but the chairman of the financially-stressed airline orders him to suck it up and make it work with 60,000 regardless, if he wants to keep his job. Now, would you want to fly with an airline like that?"

"No way!"

"Well, Will, that's the model of modern nursing! That's the way we were managing our floors, and the way we were hamstringing the most important operational asset in this whole healthcare structure: the working nurse. That's the way most hospitals in this nation are still doing it today, nurturing trouble, feeding the nursing shortage and massive turnover rates and a hundred other negative effects simply because the guys and gals at the top can't hear the voices from below. Those silent voices come from the very people on whom patient satisfaction and patient safety depends, right there at the bedside!"

"So what did you do? I'm seeing some very unique things here, but expanded nursing staffs require funding."

"What did we do? We turned the system upside down. One unit at a time, we gave the power and the responsibility to the nurses."

"I don't understand. Power to do what? Help set the staffing plan?"

She laughed. "No, Will, way beyond that, and you, as an alpha-male leader with a CEO background are *not* going to like this, but it's the only method that works. We gave all staffing authority to the charge nurse and the nurses on the floor."

"You *what*?"

"That's right. We took our best charge nurses and educated them and trained them in the new philosophy we were about to deploy. We asked them to be the stewards of our resources, and of patient safety and service quality. We asked them to staff the floor hour-by-hour as they saw fit, and we gave them all the tools and authority to do just that. We have no grids, no specified number of nurses, and no interference from above. Things change at least every four hours, and any nurse can immediately get more help when he or she needs it, or go to the float pool when things are quiet."

"How did you avoid breaking the bank? If I'd given my nurses everything they wanted in the way of additional help, they would have bankrupted us in a fortnight."

"It might have broken the bank if you changed things all at once, but not the way we did it. Even without knowing your people or the surrounding community your hospital was in, I can tell you that when you empower and educate and elevate members of an oppressed class — which describes nursing — and when you then make them responsible for the castle that they, too, depend on and work in, they seldom disappoint. I think if you'd applied the same methods you would have realized the same results we have."

"But Patti, there has to be budgetary responsibility."

"And there is. Let me give you a startling fact. After 18 months of implementing this empowerment model, we're spending almost exactly what we were spending before the changeover on nursing salaries and associated expenses and benefits, yet our patient satisfaction scores are through the roof."

"I know satisfaction's incredibly high. That's one of the reasons I'm here," he said. "But it's a *wash*? *Financially*?"

"Will, we were spending all our time and energy repairing

the old system. I think it was Buckminster Fuller who said, 'If you want to fix a system, build a new system that makes the old one outdated.'"

"I remember that quote."

"What we then did is, we shared all the financials with our front-line nurses, who, once we pulled them away from the whirlwind they'd been living in, were able to focus with great clarity on what system changes needed to be made to provide safe, quality care. There were many, many brainstorming sessions on how to economize appropriately without hurting their ability to concentrate on the patient. *They* figured out clever ways to save money, such as better ways of handling linens and supplies, and they also came up with highly effective ways of reducing nosocomial infections, which is especially important now that the government has decided that the cost of curing such infections should be borne by the hospital that caused them. Codes are down, infections are down, wasted time is down, *falls* are down, and morale is through the roof. And you know one of the main reasons why our nurses are so happy? Because we've empowered them to spend the majority of their time with their patients, at the bedside, instead of forcing them to race around eight to ten miles per day bouncing from room to room dealing with system interruptions with no time to even visit the bathroom. Anita Tucker was the researcher who verified 8.3 system interruptions per eight hour shift, and Patricia Ebright chronicled 17 per shift in 2007."[31,32]

"Okay, my head's spinning a little and I'm stuck on the financials. Let me make sure I understand this. You're telling me that when you gave the charge nurses the ability to add nurses on their floors whenever they needed them, they *didn't* rack up a, say, 40 to 60 percent increase?"

"They racked up an increase, yes, but it was below 20 percent. And, thanks to the nurse turnover rate dropping through the floor and decreased sick time and overtime, the increase was neutralized."

"You're referring to money saved from not training new nurses?"

"We peg the cost of hiring and training one new nurse at

about 80,000 dollars. Imagine the costs in a 240-bed hospital churning nurses at the rate of 50 percent per year! Even 20 percent per year. I'll show you our figures later, but we saved bundles by slashing the turnover rate, and it almost completely offset the additional costs, including the costs of physically redoing the rooms into snazzy suites."

"Amazing."

"Don't forget, Will, with dynamic, unit-based control of staffing, we can also save money by not overstaffing at slow points. Nonlinear challenge, non-linear solution. And, from the patient safety aspect, the heightened on-site scrutiny of our patients that our nurses can now provide has also sharply lowered the probability of medication and other errors leaking through, especially from harried nurses working without relief. Frankly, if you eliminate the costs of dealing with one severely injured or dead patient, I promise you'll pay for a program like this for 10 years with change left over."

Will was shaking his head and smiling the type of smile one gives to an Evel Knievel. "Jack's even braver than I thought."

"Oh, he pushed back all right, and hard. After all, with due respect to you physicians, Jack is a doctor, and despite his enlightened nature — which I'm sure you two share — he was still influenced heavily by the medical culture. You guys and gals simply have no training or experience in what nurses really do and how they do it, and what you do pick up you acquire by osmosis. The challenges facing nurses are invisible to physicians, and in Jack's case, handing over the hospital checkbook to a class of folks he didn't quite trust was frightening."

"I'm not sure trust is the right word."

"Well, I'm sure Jack had some sleepless nights. I'll also tell you more about our incredible doctor-nurse relationships here in a minute. But one more point first. Previous management had forced the nurses to unionize for their own protection. And the union thought it was doing the right thing by fighting for certain numbers and ratios. You know, so many nurses versus so many patients. But such numbers are now meaningless at St. Michael's, because whatever the workload, the nurses have the power to make their own direct decisions at the point of care, which is how we came to ditch the institution of the private room."

"Yes, how *did* you decide to do that, and why? Isn't there huge patient resistance?"

"You'd think so, but the answer is no, mainly because we did a good job explaining ourselves to our community, and they got it."

"You advertised?"

"Yes. Intensively."

"What was the hook, so to speak?"

"The TV commercial was really good. First, a patient is shown waking up with a start and ringing and ringing for a nurse while a rogue elephant tromps around her private room trumpeting and knocking over things like her flowers and an infusion machine. A nurse finally tries to answer, but she's half a building away and they can't understand each other over the intercom. The interchange is really funny, the patient yells 'Elephant!' and the nurse says 'I can't elevate you any more!' Then it cuts suddenly to the same patient waking up the same way, but this time sans elephant. She picks up what looks like the same type of remote, but instead of punching it, she just says, 'Nurse?' The shot pulls back to show our gal is just a few feet away and getting up from her console to respond. She's had a terrible dream. There's no elephant in that room. But as they're talking about it, the camera pulls back revealing the outside hallway and you see two cops escorting an elephant away. The tagline? 'Why ring for your nurse when she's five feet away? St. Michael's has a better idea.'"

"That does sound funny, and expensive."

"It was well worth it. But you asked how we made the decision. We sat our nurses down in numerous meetings, face-to-face, and said essentially this: Our core values, especially for nursing at the bedside, are safety, quality, dignity, respect, compassion and caring. Under those principles, and doing what you do best as nurses who entered the profession to care for people, what can we do to change the system for the better?"

"And they said 'wards?'"

"You're getting hung up on that word, Will. No, they didn't say 'wards' because many of them weren't old enough to even remember the concept. What they said was, 'Give us more time with our patients!' What they said was, 'How can we care for our patients when we can't even linger long enough in one room to have a decent conversation without ignoring another patient in another room who's ringing for something, or crashing, or just looking bad?' So we laid out the entire concept of a hospital floor and started punching through and throwing away all the known paradigms, and what came out of that was someone remembering a brilliant idea that the author of a series of nursing books, a nurse herself, came up with: Put the nurse in the room with her patient, only make it a room with four or five patients.[33] When you do that, two things happen that are marvelous. One — and studies solidly support this — patients get better when they're not cut off and isolated. To the patient, a hospital feels like a prison. And two, even with five patients, their nurse is right there at all times, and the guardian for each of them in almost a mother lion sort of way."

"And that's what's driven the satisfaction scores into orbit?"

"For the nurses as well as the patients. I can't tell you what a happy revolution it's been, and who knows how many accidents and incidents and falls, and even psychological meltdowns we've avoided by that constant contact. But there's a lot more!"

"Why Nurse Miller, you're almost bouncing!"

"I get very enthusiastic! No apologies."

"None required."

"Okay, here's the deal. We also found, much to our surprise, that we were charting our lives away."

"Putting too much information in the charts runs a heightened legal risk, in other words?"

"No, no, no — nothing to do with liability. But we were spending up to 23 percent of our time as nurses, that's from a national study, charting things that no one read, no one needed, and that accomplished nothing.[34] It was CYA charting! The docs never read our notes. Heck, Will, *we* didn't read our notes."

"I guess I've always known that."

"There's a great cartoon from the *New Yorker* of a few years back featuring a distinguished man stopping in downtown New York to read the words on an elaborate brass plaque. 'On this precise location on April 12, 1796,' it says, 'absolutely nothing at all happened.' That's the story of our charting. In fact, there are only two federal charting requirements, notes that involve restraints and follow-ups on pain."

"You didn't stop charting, though?"

"We instituted a major change and now we chart by exception. We document what changes, what goes wrong, what needs attention, not the fact that the sun comes up in the east every morning and the patient is still breathing. We identify the problem, the plan and what we're supposed to do. That's it. And our doctors actually read it. In fact *everyone* reads the notes because they get to the point and contain vital information, not station-keeping chronicles. Now, where the charting once served as a poor checklist (I've checked this, I've checked that) we use individual checklists for tracking our personal work sequence, and floor checklists for specific duties and procedures. We've designed those as a group for standardization."

"Did you use any patient focus groups, or anything similar?"

"We sure did. We asked patients who'd been here in the previous year what they valued most, and they said trusting the staff and feeling safe, and knowing they could talk to their nurse when they needed something. Patients are aware these days that there's a huge patient safety problem, and they're coming in here now trying to remember what they need to guard against — look out for hand washing, bad medication — and now there's a growing understanding, if you will, that a hospital is not an inherently safe place. But there's also not enough education for a patient or the patient's family and friends to feel secure in knowing what to look out for. So we invented something new that has worked wonderfully — the patient safety coach. Not like the patient safety coaching of staff, though. These are people who coach the patient and family exclusively. We started with just one person in the position and now have two. When someone's admitted, we start them and their family out with a really great video.[35] It's very frank, it's essentially done by us, and it tells the patient and the family that they are an integral part of our patient safety system, and they need to understand how to be fully engaged. We talk about the fact that it's a complex human system, and we give them the details about who to talk to and when. Then the patient safety coach introduces himself or herself and works on making sure they really are engaged, which helps allay their fears at the same time it helps them accept their responsibilities as patients. That has all sorts of benefits, including gaining a greater degree of cooperation even after discharge. We've also introduced bedside bar-coding, and it's a zero-exceptions system, short of a code. We also established a no-interruption zone around each Pixus and an actual signal — a red towel we throw over our left shoulder when we're drawing, administering, or otherwise dealing with medications — that is inviolable. You do not ever interrupt a nurse with a red towel on her or his shoulder, unless there's a code or a fire. Period. And now that we're making the transition to computer records, the change we've already made is working even better."

"Tell me how you came up with the design of the rooms? Are they all exactly like the one I saw?"

"We have three basic types of five-bedroom suites, with the number of windows being the variable. The individual roomettes radiate out from a central point, which is the nurses' desk. Each roomette can be separated along the side from the others, and a curtain pulled for complete visual privacy, but most of the time the nurse can watch all five beds at once and can hear her patients. As I said, we don't need call lights and worries about response times because the nurse is right there with her patients, constantly. And what we also did with this overhaul was realize that all the hoo-hah about pretending a hospital room was a first-class hotel with a five-star restaurant is nonsense. Plan to visit a five-star *after* you get out of the hospital. This isn't a hotel, it's an environment in which we do our best to make you get better as fast as reasonably possible, and help you feel as comfortable as possible in the meantime. And, we banished the word 'customer.' It was irritating all of us anyway. When you're admitted to St. Michael's, you're not a customer, you're our patient. A patient has a far higher status than a customer. Now, should we still strive to serve good food and have a reasonable selection available? Of course, but that should never take precedent over the care we provide, and it was doing just that. The tail was wagging the dog, and we were beginning to forget what our purpose was."

"Wow. You've taken a harpoon to just about everything."

"Well, not everything. But we've changed a lot. Oh, and another thing. We put pedometers on our nurses before we made the changes, which is why we know that some were hiking around eight miles per shift. Absolute horrible inefficiency, and if it hadn't been for the stress all that bouncing around created, we might have dubbed it a thinly disguised physical fitness program. But it had to change, and boy has it. By decentralizing supplies and even medications, we've cut waste as well as unnecessary trips."

"Decentralized? How?"

"The supplies are at the bedside now, right in the rooms. Each room — or suite, if you like — has a Pixus at the nurse's console that opens with the nurse's thumbprint. In other words, we now bring the point of supply to the point of care. That little electronic controller you saw Jan handing off to Claire a while ago that looked like a sophisticated universal remote?"

"The handheld device with the screen?"

"Yes. It's connected wirelessly to a small device the patient has. The patient programs in what his or her maximum pain tolerance is, and then every hour it flashes and beeps to remind the patient to punch in whatever number corresponds with their current pain level, in a sort of instant report. That pops up on the portable device and is recorded automatically in the electronic chart. If the reported pain level is at or above the maximum the patient recorded, it goes into alarm and we're there instantly, and the patient can enter a special report at any time. There's another button on the patient's device for mobility, so if their nurse is at the far corner of the room or they don't want to raise their voice, punching the button does the job. Most of the time, though, a patient just speaks up in a normal voice and is heard immediately."

"Next you'll tell me there's an exam table that reads all parameters without touching the patient, *Star Trek*-style."

"We're working on it, actually. Technology has not historically made the nurses' job any easier. But I'm not through, Will. Did you notice our LPNs?"

"Yes."

"Okay, there's one RN for each suite, and at least one LPN to assist for baths and anything else needed. We don't hire two-year degree RNs any more, by the way. We grandfathered in our two-year degree RNs, of course, but we require them to get a four-year degree and help them do so, and we expect our four-year RNs to all earn master's degrees within five years. Education minimizes the power imbalance."

"Impressive. Jack said you'd taken some action regarding the varying nursing degrees."

"That disparity has got to be halted nationwide. The training to get to RN has to be finite and the same across the country. In fact, we're hard at work at, and really excited about, the idea of changing the normal four year curriculum for an RN degree to include full qualification as a physician's assistant. We think the legislature is going to go along with us, and after all, today's nurse desperately needs the same abilities to issue and modify medication orders as PA's possess."

"Patti, what was the biggest 'Aha!' for the administration? For Jack and the board?"

She smiled and studied the wall for a few moments, composing the words. "It was more of an 'Oh my gosh!' than an 'Aha,' Will. Jack and the board feared that handing over any degree of power would constitute letting the inmates run the asylum. It was mostly an unconscious fear, but it was huge, and when the nurses *didn't* run away with the treasury and didn't misuse their power, Jack and the board were all but stunned. We calmed them down by making this a pilot study — starting with one floor at a time. Now, I think the second 'Aha!' was there, too, and that had to do with the concept that our most important focus was safe, quality care. I know they really believed it was true. But after these changes took effect, Jack was honest enough to say he was also stunned to discover that the most important focus for the board had always been the finances."

"And the biggest "Aha!' for the nurses?"

"That staffing wasn't our primary problem, as we had always believed. We'd never seen beyond the staffing issues. We hyperventilated over them every day, but once that bogeyman was gone, we suddenly began to see the incredible waste and the galaxy of workarounds and the incredibly unsafe attitudes and behaviors that had all been invisible when we thought the only problem was the numbers of us per patient."

"Really? It was that dramatic?"

"Will, I'd guess 90 percent of America's hospitals would experience exactly the same thing as soon as the staffing issue disappeared. Suddenly it all seemed so straightforward, and our metrics prove it."

He sat back, shaking his head in admiration. "Incredible, Patti. You've created quite a flagship here."

"Flagship is an interesting word. You mean, as in an example for the rest of health care, right?"

"Exactly."

"We're not a template or a hard-and-fast example to be duplicated on each point, Will. Focus on the concepts, which are a refocus of priorities, not tactics. The point is patient care, and when we make that number one, we can solve all the other problems. The key element is empowering the people at the bedside and letting them light the way to the specific tactical changes. The same process may lead to different solutions in other hospitals, but the key is in redesigning the entire medical center to serve the patient's best interests, and you do that by redesigning the hospital as an entity to *support* the nurses and the doctors. You know, the sharp end of the system used to be the problem. We've made it the solution, and therein lies the method that can change every hospital in America."

She looked at her watch, then back at Will. "Your choice, but would you like to tour around up here a bit more, just sit and observe in one of the suites, or head on out? I've got one of our senior surgeons due in tomorrow morning for what we call a follow day, but I could set one up for you, too."

"A 'follow day?'"

"We require each of our doctors to follow a nurse around for an entire shift once per year."

"How do they have the time?"

"They don't have the time not to. It's a cornerstone of our interdisciplinary, anti-silo efforts."

Will shook his head. "Frankly, I'd love to do that, or at least spend the rest of the day watching the incredible interplays you've set up here, but I've got a flight to catch, and I promised Jack to drop back by before I left."

"Fair enough," she said, handing him her card. "Please call my secretary any time for any follow-up information, or if you'd like to come spend some time on the floor. I left a packet of internal papers in Jack's office for you on all of this, including some of the working papers we used to design the suites."

"Your secretary?" Will said surprised.

"Yes Will. When we looked at our manager workload there were a host of changes as well, but the first one was the realization that we spent the majority of our time in our office making telephone calls for staffing, filing, paperwork, etcetera. We belong with the patients, doctors and staff — NOT behind closed doors trying to direct quality from an invisible command post."

He shook her hand and thanked her as she pointed him back down the corridor toward the elevator.

"Don't forget what I said, Will."

"Which part?" He laughed.

"About getting back in the saddle after falling off the horse."

"Excuse me?"

"Being a CEO again."

Will's Notes:

The changes St. Michael's has pioneered in nursing are mind-boggling! First, the Suites, the position of the nurses station IN each suite with its own Pixus; the way they conduct their "reports," their charting by exception methods, and perhaps most amazing, the fact that the hospital has turned over all the staffing authority to the nurses themselves, resulting in the major financial benefit of achieving a reduction in the turnover rate. In addition, they openly advertised the new multiple-bed rooms (suites) and have received strong public support.

They use a Patient Safety Coach to indoctrinate every newly admitted patient and family/friends, along with a well-produced video outlining the patient/family responsibilities and how to interface with the nursing and physician staff.

Bedside bar-coding is used throughout with no-exceptions, other than codes.

Concept of the "No Interruption Zone" extends to any nurse drawing up medication or just getting it out of a Pixus.

They use a patient-programmed pain tolerance instrument and the nurse carries what looks like a universal remote with a screen, but it tells her all the pain med settings of her patients and any immediate needs they trigger.

CHAPTER FIFTEEN

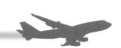

The usual busy day was unfolding at St. Michael's Hospital as Will put the rental car in gear, then returned the shift lever to park, giving himself a few more minutes to study the place from across the parking lot. The overstuffed folder of information Jack had compiled included Patti's packet, all of it now weighing down the passenger seat beside him. The last 20 minutes of conversation with St. Michael's CEO had covered the changes in some of the departments he hadn't had time to visit directly. All of it, Will thought, had provided a far more comprehensive tour than he'd had any right to expect.

But it had been something Jack said as they walked to the door that wouldn't let him go.

"Will, the obstacle you tried unsuccessfully to deal with 10 years ago proved unmovable because most of it was unseen. Like an iceberg showing only the top 10 percent, these challenges are monumental and far deeper than any of us once thought. You were trying to move that iceberg, Will, with a rowboat, and you were almost certain to fall without the proper equipment and understanding of the problem. You did your best, and keep in mind that for dynamic people, there truly is a path to self-forgiveness, and you need to find that path."

He'd let it slide past in that moment, not entirely sure what Jack meant. But now, in the glaring light of hindsight and with all he'd seen and learned in the past three days, the ultimate futility of what he'd tried to accomplish as a hospital CEO was painfully apparent. The best of intentions and energy and effort had been hobbled by the inertia of tradition, and it had defeated his grand vision of a thoroughly safe medical center, killing his godson in the process. He could see that now. But what, exactly, had Jack meant that there was a path to self-forgiveness?

Will grimaced as the events of that night passed through his mind yet again. The logical side of him — the left-brain matrix of thought — had long since reported in detail on all the opportunities that had been missed that could have saved young Ronnie. None of those lost chances had resulted from dereliction of duty or negligence, but from institutional ignorance of what it would have taken to make his hospital as safe as he'd thought it was. That reality now shook the foundation of his self-imposed guilt, even though the right side of his cerebral cortex wanted to refuse the logic and cling to the painful reality that the loss had occurred on his watch and a solemn trust had been breached.

But that, too, was beginning ever so slightly to change. If he were to hold himself accountable, after all he'd seen at St. Michael's, it should be for not knowing how to break through calcified communications barriers and build truly collegial teams, for not understanding the tremendous pressure that comes from "That's the way we've always done it," and for not knowing how to truly maximize power in his organization. Perhaps that was Jack's point: that understanding led to self-forgiveness. He would need to think on that.

Will slipped the car in gear again and motored out toward the Interstate, the course to Denver International already memorized. Janice, his wife of 18 years, would be meeting him on the other end at the airport, and while he'd given her a headline news sketch of what he was learning, he knew she was still mystified by what he thought he was accomplishing in spending three days away from his clinic. He hadn't been able to articulate then, and probably couldn't now, why it was so important to find out what he hadn't known. It just was.

Various snippets of conversation from the past three days played in his mind as he dropped the car at the rental lot and rode the bus to the terminal, aware that he was once again suppressing the same old feeling of hopelessness. He was holding his boarding pass and waiting for his row to be called when his cell phone rang, and he had to fumble a bit to open the device and punch it on.

"Hello?"

"Will, Jack Silverman. One last thought."

"Sure, Jack. I'm just getting ready to board."

"Can you take down a number?"

"Ah... hang on." More fumbling produced a notebook and pen. "Okay. Go ahead."

Jack passed a phone number and an unfamiliar name.

"And, what should I do with Mr. Mason's name and number, Jack?"

"Well, turns out Mason may have something you need."

The voice of the gate agent boomed overhead on the PA drowning out even his thoughts for a second.

"Those of you holding boarding passes for Zone three are now welcome to board. Zones one through three."

"Sorry, Jack. That PA was loud enough to be heard in Zanzibar. You were saying?"

"Mason's a good man, and in my humble opinion, he has a key to your puzzle."

"My puzzle?"

"Will, you came to us looking for ways to make patient safety really take off and stay where we want it, in the stratosphere. Am I right?"

"Yes."

"Well, let's stick to the aviation metaphor. He's got the plane but no pilot; you're a pilot with no plane. And we just invested three days teaching you how to fly a hospital."

"Jack, you're talking in parables."

"Okay, try this. He's the board chairman of a 200-bed facility in Las Vegas that's melting down. He needs a CEO, and you need a second chance. Give the man a call, Dr. Jenkins. Make us proud."

EPILOGUE

It is very difficult to patch and rebuild a leaking ship while you're sailing it, yet that is exactly the magnitude of the challenge faced by American medicine. In fact, the status quo IS sinking the ship, especially with respect to the fact that after nine years of concerted effort to reduce patient risk from medical mistakes, we have barely moved the needle. Why so little measurable success? Because this quest involves nothing less than massive cultural change, and that takes years of sustained, coordinated and focused effort. In effect, we're at the beginning of the journey.

The focus, however, constitutes much of the problem. Heretofore, it's been all over the map. As one of the founding board members of the National Patient Safety Foundation who stuck with the foundation for nine years hoping against frustration that we could finally construct and install the solutions, I can tell you that the propensity of all of us in this fight is to hop on our horses and ride off in all directions. From instituting forcing functions to computerization, through instituting checklists and read-backs, and a hundred other protocols, healthcare professionals (with the help of NPSF, IHI, Leapfrog, the Joint Commission and specifically the IOM) have succeeded in massively raising awareness of the depth of the patient safety crisis and the challenges of even reaching a common definition of quality. But, there has been no unifying success in simply painting the vision of what it would all look like working together in harmony. And one of the prime reasons for that is that we fell victim once again to our very American propensity to dehumanize even our most human of institutions: We forget about the impact on the people who ARE healthcare and their patients and patient's families, and what it's like for them on a daily basis.

The business of medical practice — contemporarily short-handed as "Healthcare" — is alive with ongoing and noble attempts by dedicated people to overhaul the system in order to make it both highly reliable and high-quality. The daunting barriers, however, include a combination of inertia (This is the way we've always done it), cottage industry/farmer's market structure (You can't tell me what to do, I don't work for your hospital), and the fact that we insist on thinking of healthcare as an industry instead of America's most vital public utility. Within these realities, it is my strong belief that without a model of what a successful, safe, and yes, reasonably happy hospital looks like — *and feels like* — all these thousands of individual efforts have no overall focus. That's the reason for "constructing" St. Michael's in this book — to provide a beginning aim point.

And let me hammer away at that one concept, the idea of what a high-reliability, high-quality institution FEELS like to the people who not only work there, but who ARE that institution. If we don't put the major emphasis on how the doctors and nurses and pharmacists and managers feel about their work and their relationships with each other, we haven't a prayer of plugging the holes that have been sinking the ship.

Ultimately, the root cause of the problems that bedevil us is the "business model" of American healthcare. In a simple phrase, it's wired backwards. As George Halvorson points out in *Healthcare Reform Now!*, out of thousands of billing codes for thousands of medical services, there is not a single one for "wellness," or keeping patients in good health, which, of course, is the ultimate goal of every doctor and nurse and participant. That's not a moral failure, it's a structural failure, and it bespeaks the desperate need for a national "moonshot" focus led by whoever sits in the Oval Office dedicating us to completely redesign the engine of the ship in ways that directly reward medical people and institutions for creating health. Today, doing the right thing and minimizing the use of medical services by improving health means less revenue and an inherent penalty. We have to change that equation drastically. Interestingly enough, the best method of doing that may ultimately resemble more of a mechanical engineering solution than a complex financial and governmental structure, and — as my fictional CEO Jack Silverman says in this book — it may revolve more around community-based funding methods than any national solution. But however we rewire it — and while virtually all of American healthcare needs to be thinking hard about how to achieve this very obvious and yet very ignored goal — we have to start with the present crisis. We must reverse the reality that there are few places as potentially dangerous to human life and welfare (from mistakes) as the American hospital.

My St. Michael's in this book is neither a perfect hospital model nor the ultimate one. It is, however, a place where the majority of the great ideas and human realities can be viewed together — ideas which have been whirling around this community in fragmented fashion before and after the IOM's pivotal report of 1999 (as well as their follow-on 2001 report, *Crossing the Quality Chasm*). St. Michael's is a beginning ideal, and having an ideal is vital if we are to focus that same dynamic American energy that has won wars, gone to the moon, and created a can-do societal attitude that knows no bounds.

John J. Nance, JD

ENDNOTES

1. Comparison formulated by Spence Bynum, Managing Partner, Convergent HRS, LLC, 2007.

2. Dixon, NM, Shofer, M: Patterns, culture, and reliability: Struggling to invent high-reliability organizations in health care settings: Insights from the field. Health Research and Educational Trust (*Health Service Res*), Aug 2006; 41(4 pt.2): 1618-32.

3. Some of the more important contributing causes at Tenerife included:

   - The hierarchical culture of the cockpit that intimidated subordinate crewmembers from speaking up when time-critical problems arose about which they were uncertain.

   - The cultural presumption that senior leaders were significantly less capable of error than less experienced subordinates (The Halo Effect).

   - The garbled radio communications resulting from inadequate discipline in the use of Aviation English as a standard, the defined and taught international language of aviation air traffic control.

   - The limitations of using a single radio frequency in which only one radio at a time can transmit, and through which only a finite amount of information can be transmitted in a given period of time.

   - The fuel requirements and procedures that contributed to the captain's decision to refuel at Tenerife instead of Las Palmas.

- The captain's failure to assure that he had received a takeoff clearance.

- The first officer's acceptance of a clearly inadequate take-off "clearance" and his assumption that it was sufficient.

- The airline's failure to authorize and direct even second officers to order an aborted takeoff when something seems seriously wrong or questionable.

- The absence of anything approaching crew coordination training at KLM (or any airline at that time) dictating that all crewmembers be fully engaged in critical decisions, including takeoff in foggy conditions.

- The use of Tenerife as an alternate airport when Las Palmas was closed.

4. Leape, LL, Brennan, TA, Laird, NM, et al. The nature of adverse events in hospitalized patients: Results from the Harvard Medical Practice Study II. *New Engl J. Med*, 1991, 324:377-384.

5. Brennan, TA, Leape LL, Laird NM, et al. Incidence of adverse events and negligence in hospitalized patients: Results from the Harvard Medical Practice Study I. *New Engl J. Med*, 1991, 324:370-376.

6. Capra F: *The Web of Life*. Anchor Books, New York, NY, 1996

7. Amazingly enough, this is a true story with the names and locale changed.

8. Rosenstein AH: Nurse-physician relationships: impact on nurse satisfaction and retention. *American Journal of Nursing*, Vol. 102(6), June 2002, pp 26-34.

9. Rosenstein AH, O'Daniel M: Disruptive behavior and clinical outcomes: Nurses and physicians. *American Journal of Nursing*, Vol. 105(1), January 2005, pp 54-64.

10. *Ending Nurse-to-Nurse Hostility: Why Nurses Eat Their Young and Each Other*. Bartholomew KM, HCPro, Marblehead, MA, 2006.

11. *Speak your Truth: Proven Strategies for Effective Nurse-Physician Communication.* Bartholomew KM, HCPro, Marblehead, MA, 2005.

12. See Heparin Overdose Deaths of Infants Linked to Mistaken Stocking of Automated Pharmacy Dispensers. Web article requires registration for site but may be found at "http://-/pt.wkhealth.com/pt/re/nbs/abstract.00149078-200610150-00013.htm;jsessionid=Hr2WwqqL1wm1tyS2Rq91vZWRwX pgjGHh66Ynd264h9qhTNh0gMKw!1138671057!18119562 9!8091!-1;" *Patient Week Health*; 36(18):143, October 15, 2006; staff article.

13. Ornstein C, Gorman A: Dennis Quaid's newborns reportedly harmed by medical mixup. *Los Angeles Times*, November 27, 2007. Web citation at: http://www.latimes.com/news/local/la-me-twins21nov21,1,5462484.story?coll=la-headlines-california 2007.

14. Gurses AP, Carayon P: Performance obstacles of intensive care nurses. *Nursing Research*, 2007, May-Jun, 56(3), 185-194.

15. Jain M, Miller L, Belt D, King D, Berwick DM: Decline in ICU adverse events: Nosocomial infections and cost through a quality improvement initiative focusing on teamwork and culture change. *Quality Safety Healthcare*, August 2006, 15(4): 235-9.

16. *Healthcare Reform Now!: A Prescription for Change.* Halvorson GC, John Wiley & Sons, San Francisco, CA, 2007. From page 73, paragraph 2, "If we are going to systematically improve care and recognize when care is not being delivered at acceptable levels, we need real, current, and appropriate data. The best source of that data is the full automated electronic medical record."

17. Aviation Safety Reporting System run by NASA, Moffet Field, California; Web address: http://asrs.arc.nasa.gov/.

18. Bagian JP, Lee C, Gosbee J, DeRosier J, et al: Developing and deploying a patient safety program in a large health care delivery system: you can't fix what you don't know about.

Joint Commission Journal of Quality Improvement, Oct. 2001; 27(10):522-32.

19. NTSB Aircraft Accident Report AAR/92-02, 1.17.1 at pp 57.

20. Milch CE, Salem DN, Pauker SG, Lundquist TG, Kumar S, Chen J; Department of Medicine and the Institute for Clinical Research and Health Policy Studies, Tufts-New England Medical Center, Boston, MA; *Voluntary electronic reporting of medical errors and adverse events. An analysis of 92,547 reports from 26 acute-care hospitals.* J Gen Intern Med. 2006 Feb; 21(2): 165-70. Epub Dec 22, 2005.

21. Furman C, Caplan R: Applying the Toyota Production System: Using a patient safety alert system to reduce error: *Joint Commission Journal of Quality and Patient Safety*; July 2007; 33(7):376-86, With reference to Virginia Mason Medical Center's pioneering efforts in Seattle, Wash. "As of December 2006, 6,112 Patient Safety Alert (PSA) reports were received: 20% from managers, 8% from physicians, 44% from nurses, and 23% from non-clinical support personnel..." "Discussion: Implementing the PSA system has drastically increased the number of safety concerns that are resolved at VMMC, while drastically reducing the time it takes to resolve them. Transparent discussion and feedback have helped promote staff acceptance and participation."

22. *The Challenger Launch Decision.* Vaughn, D; University of Chicago Press, 1996.

23. Bartholomew, KM: *Ending Nurse-to-Nurse Hostility.* ibid.

24. *First, Do No Harm.* Produced by the Partnership for Patient Safety, P4PS: One West Superior Street, Suite 2410, Chicago, IL 60610; Web Address: http://www.p4ps.org/interactive_videos.asp

25. See National Transportation Safety Board Docket # DCA06MA064. See also Web address citation: http://ntsb.gov/ntsb/brief.asp?ev_id=20060828X01244&key=1.

26. "The Global War on Error" is a registered trademark of Dr. Anthony Kern. Dr. Kern is the CEO of Convergent Knowledge Solutions, which may be reached through (703) 441-9213, cks411@convergent-knowledge.com, or their website at http://www.convergent-knowledge.com.

27. Arnedt, JT, Wilde, GJS, Munt, PW et al: How do prolonged wakefulness and alcohol compare in the decrements they produce on a simulated driving task. *Accident Analysis and Prevention* 2001, 33(3), 47-54.

28. Convergent Knowledge Solutions may be reached through: cks411@convergent-knowledge.com, or their website at http://www.convergent-knowledge.com.

29. *The Culture Code*. Rapaille, C; Broadway Books, New York, NY, 2006, p. 82.

30. See NTSB Accident Report AAR-92-02. A non-official transcript of the Cockpit Voice Recorder may be downloaded from www.WhyHospitalsShouldFly.com.

31. Operational failures and interruptions in hospital nursing; Tucker AL; Spear SJ; *Health Serv Res*, 2006 June;41(3 Pt 1): 643-62.

32. Ebright PR; Patterson ES; Chalko BA; Render ML: Understanding the complexity of registered nurse work in acute care settings; *Journal of Nursing Administration*, (2003), 33(12),630-638.

33. While various forms of patient suites are already in operation in various hospitals, this specific plan was devised by Kathleen Bartholomew (See *Ending Nurse-to-Nurse Hostility and Speak Your Truth*, ibid), after studying the dynamics of nurse-to-patient ratios, communication barriers and extensive experience with the physical limitations single rooms impose on the ability of nurses to provide focused personal care.

34. Potter P, Wolf L, Boxerman S, et al: Understanding the cognitive work of nursing in the acute care environment. *JONA*, Vol 35,7/8,pp 327-335 (2005) at 329 col 2.

35. Such videos have been developed at several institutions using the template set forth by the Joint Commission. Assistance on producing such a video can be found at www.WhyHospitalsShouldFly.com.

ACKNOWLEDGMENTS

There are a host of dedicated medical professionals who assisted in the preparation and proofing of this work, and without question the most important is the person to whom it is dedicated, Kathleen Bartholomew, RN, MN—the author of three books and perhaps the most important contributor today in the quest of rescuing and reviving the profession of nursing.

Special thanks also goes to Cathy Whitaker, RN, MBA, whose superb guidance on which voice to use in energizing hospital leaders while reaching the entirety of healthcare was right on the mark.

In addition, I deeply appreciate the early comments and counsel of Dr. Diana Kramer of Seattle, who read an early version of the manuscript. Her insights were invaluable in keeping the balance of the message equally resonant with physicians.

I also appreciate very much the detailed read and important suggestions provided by Dr. John Byrnes and Dr. Jim Reinertsen, as well as the enthusiasm and feedback afforded by John-Henry Pfifferling, Ph.D., of Durham, North Carolina; Elaine Goehner, RN, of Seattle; Captain James J. Nance of Loveland, Colorado; and my daughter, Bridgitte Krupke of Culver City, California, a visual effects producer and consummate professional photographer who shot the cover picture of her dad.

I am deeply indebted to Dr. David Nash, Professor and Chair of the Department of Health Policy at Jefferson Medical College, who wrote the Foreword; Dr. Lucian Leape of the Harvard School of Public Health, who penned the Introduction; and Dr. Don Berwick, President of the Institute for Healthcare Improvement, for his gracious endorsement, as well as the fellow founding board members of the National Patient Safety Foundation who agreed to read and comment on the manuscript. Any contributions that don't make it in time for the first edition will be prominently featured on the website WhyHospitalsShouldFly.com, which I intend to be a living and constantly changing support forum for this work and the model it seeks to create.

Finally, and perhaps most importantly, I want to express my deep appreciation to my team in Bozeman, Montana, at Second River Healthcare Press—the publishing house that is rapidly becoming a substantial force in healthcare information. Even as a veteran of 18 internationally published books, I was amazed at the hands-on support and teamwork of Jerry Pogue, my Publisher (who is a visionary and highly experienced former hospital CEO) and my Editor, Chris Jackson, both of whom set new standards in redefining collegiality and the concept of the common goal. Frankly, they provide a living, breathing model for the best of what publishers used to be, and could be again.

ABOUT THE AUTHOR

John J. Nance, JD has been a dynamic and deeply dedicated member of the medical community for nearly two decades. Speaker, consultant and best selling author, John brings a rich diversity of professional training and background to the quest of patient safety and medical practice improvement. His new book, *Why Hospitals Should Fly: The Ultimate Flight Plan to Patient Safety and Quality Care* (Second River Healthcare Press 2008), is reinventing the cultural foundations of healthcare and bringing clarity to the decade-long patient safety and quality care debate.

John was one of the founding members of the National Patient Safety Foundation and a member of the Executive Committee who served on the board for 9 years. He is a native Texan who grew up in Dallas where he earned his Bachelor's Degree from Southern Methodist University (SMU) and his Juris Doctor Degree from SMU School of Law before admission to the Texas bar. Installed as a Distinguished Alumni of Southern Methodist University in 2002, he is also a decorated Air Force officer-pilot veteran of Vietnam and Operations Desert Storm/Desert Shield, and a Lt. Colonel in the USAF Reserve, well known for his pioneering involvement in Air Force human factors flight safety education. As a professional pilot, John has piloted a wide variety of jet aircraft, including most of Boeing's line as well as the Air Force C-141, and has logged over 13,000 hours of flight time in his commercial airline (Braniff and Alaska) and Air Force careers. But more important to his leading-edge role in healthcare, John Nance was one of the pioneers of the pivotal safety revolution in professional communication, teamwork, and leadership known in aviation as CRM, crew resource management. His book about safety in human systems entitled *BLIND TRUST*, published internationally in 1986, is widely credited with helping to spark not only the universal acceptance of CRM principles in aviation, but the earliest infusion of culture-changing lessons derived from aviation into medical practice. *BLIND TRUST* was pivotal in illuminating serious public issues in aviation safety for the American public, and *WHY HOSPITALS SHOULD FLY* follows in that tradition as a major wakeup call.

John has become a trusted and internationally recognized broadcast analyst and advocate for both medical/patient safety and aviation safety. Before joining *ABC World News* and *Good Morning America* in 1994, he had logged countless appearances on national shows such as *Oprah*, the *PBS News Hour*, *Today*, CNN, as well as most Canadian and English-speaking networks worldwide. In addition, his editorials have been published in newspapers nationwide, inclusive of the *Los Angeles Times* and *USA Today*, and he has been listed for more than a decade in *Who's Who in America*.

John J. Nance is also the internationally-known author of 18 major books (five non-fiction, 13 fiction), his latest fiction thriller being *Orbit* (Simon and Schuster) which released to rave reviews in March of 2006 and is in development by Fox 2000 studios as a major motion picture. Two other of his books, *Pandora's Clock* and *Medusa's Child*, were both made into major, successful two-part mini-series for NBC and ABC respectively, and still air periodically around the world.

With most of his busy schedule of consulting and speaking dedicated to the urgency of improving healthcare from patient safety to practice satisfaction, John has also emerged as one of the leading thinkers on matters of major change to America's healthcare system. A dynamic and vocal advocate of completely removing the tort system from involvement in routine medical accidents and mistakes, he recently convened and hosted an unprecedented conference on the subject with the sponsorship of AHRQ, a conference of doctors and lawyers that spawned several very surprising and important realizations.

Already one of the nation's most dynamic and energizing professional speakers, John J. Nance's messages to medical practitioners have reached new heights of relevance and importance as seen in his presentations to such pace-setting entities as the Institute for Healthcare Improvement and a who's who of healthcare organizations.

John's unique ability to reach every member of the healthcare community comes from his unprecedented background mix of law, safety, aviation and even broadcasting. Physicians in particular resonate deeply with his powerful messages about leadership and the human propensity for mistakes even among the most tenured professionals, and his extensive experience working with hospitals and clinics nationwide has been documented by continuous client praise and the highest effectiveness ratings.

John J. Nance lives in Seattle, Washington, and travels among healthcare organizations nationwide.

Are You Ready To Fly?

To learn more about *Why Hospitals Should Fly: The Ultimate Flight Plan to Patient Safety and Quality Care*, and John Nance's speaking and consulting services please visit:

www.WhyHospitalsShouldFly.com

If you would like to share your insights, ideas, or if you have questions for John J. Nance you can email him at:

JJN@WhyHospitalsShouldFly.com

This book is available in quantity discounts from Second River Healthcare Press. Please visit:

www.SecondRiverHealthcare.com

For personal assistance please call:

(406) 586-8775